"Like no other work of its scope and intellectual rigor, this book showcases the unique potential of hypertext to transform storytelling and narrative therapy—not only as an authoring platform and textual format, but as a method of critical inquiry, research-creation and personalized expression: A must-read for all scholars and practitioners interested in exploring and revisiting a textual practice often misunderstood and underestimated."

**Astrid Ensslin**, Professor of Digital Cultures and Communication, Director of DAS|LAB and of the Electronic Literature Organization, University of Regensburg, Germany.

# Hyperandrogenism and the Marginalization of Pathologized Bodies

In the current sociopolitical landscape, hyperandrogenism has become a lightning rod for collective anxieties about transgender identities and "preserving" women's sports, as well as misunderstandings about the inherent fairness of sport and the biological mechanisms that quantify athletic advantage. Perched behind this discourse, people living with hyperandrogenism face ongoing destabilization of healthcare access and find their experiences are often silenced and marginalized.

This book offers a novel therapeutic method for individuals with hyperandrogenism to share their experiences using literary hypertext—a form of digital storytelling that invites readers to participate by selecting hyperlinks. Focusing on a case study of women and nonbinary individuals with hyperandrogenism, ten hypertext authors' narratives are explored. Their experiences highlight the therapeutic value of writing a hypertext illness narrative by mapping reflective experiences through hyperlinks and sharing their narrative with the broader community.

Providing interdisciplinary insights into the lived experience of hyperandrogenism, as well as practical guidance on the clinical use of literary text, this book will appeal to researchers and clinicians interested in hyperandrogenism, gender studies, health humanities, narrative therapy, electronic media, game design and feminist media studies.

**Megan Perram** is an assistant professor of English at Campion College, University of Regina, Canada, specializing in digital literature and new media studies.

# Hyperandrogenism and the Marginalization of Pathologized Bodies

## Exploring Therapeutic Storytelling in Hypertext Illness Narratives

**Megan Perram**

Routledge
Taylor & Francis Group
NEW YORK AND LONDON

First published 2026
by Routledge
605 Third Avenue, New York, NY 10158

and by Routledge
4 Park Square, Milton Park, Abingdon, Oxon, OX14 4RN

*Routledge is an imprint of the Taylor & Francis Group, an informa business*



ISBN: 978-1-041-08785-4 (hbk)
ISBN: 978-1-041-08788-5 (pbk)
ISBN: 978-1-003-64692-1 (ebk)

DOI: 10.4324/9781003646921

Typeset in Times New Roman
by SPi Technologies India Pvt Ltd (Straive)

*For the ten authors who shared their stories for this work.*

# Contents

# Preface

This book theorizes the experience of hyperandrogenism, a condition that elevates androgens in the female body, through a novel therapeutic method that bridges illness narratives with hypertext. This method offers an innovative approach for those seeking accessible ways to improve well-being. In our current sociopolitical landscape, hyperandrogenism has become a global lightning rod for collective anxieties about transness and "preserving" women's sports, as well as misunderstandings about the inherent fairness of sport and the biological mechanisms that quantify athletic advantage. Perched behind this heavy discourse that is seeping into policies and legislation, there are real people living with hyperandrogenism who face ongoing destabilization of healthcare access. This book offers a way to tell our *sick* stories in clinical spaces, at the kitchen table or on a mobile device, in ways that reclaim the agency of authorship. For the afflicted at the margins, this book proposes the hyperlink.

What I hope you, the reader, take away from this work is a fresh perspective on the revelations and pitfalls of the promise of emerging technology trope. The vantage point of this book is (1) fundamentally interdisciplinary and (2) anchored by the words (and hyperlinks) of real users. This book draws from fields such as gender studies, biology, digital humanities, health humanities and narrative therapy while, at the same time, pulling from diverse methods for both conducting and presenting research findings. The Twine stories of ten authors are at the core, but they are explored in a new way. Rather than solely chronologically, textually or orally, these stories are woven together through a matrix of these and other methods, using a truly novel approach: hypertext.

The chapters of this work are theory-dense and tailored for academics; however, the manuscript shifts gears midway, offering a politicized narrative therapy-informed DIY guide to creating your own illness narrative module. This space offers a critical way for praxis to emerge—to apply the theory in accessible, real-time formats (e.g., "go here, click here"). Finally, this book is timely in every sense. It introduces a much-needed therapeutic method for marginalized people in the wake of recent and always healthcare constraints. It also engages with the ongoing public discourse surrounding the hot-button issue of "sex verification testing" in global athletics, including the Olympics, through the poorly understood condition of hyperandrogenism.

This manuscript is an original work by Megan Perram, based on a research project approved by the University of Alberta Research Ethics Board (ID Pro00098579, March 30, 2020) and revised from a PhD dissertation defended in June 2023.

Sections of this work have been previously published. A section of the first chapter within the header "A Note on Language" has been published in the 2022 article "The Possibilities of Illness Narratives in Virtual Reality for Bodies at the Margins" co-authored with Dr. Astrid Ensslin in the journal *Digital Creativity*. Small sections of Chapter 2 within the headings "Electronic Literature" and "Literary Hypertext and Rhizomatic Multiplicity" are published in a 2024 solo-authored article called "Building Hypertext Literature Reviews for Qualitative Research" in *Interdisciplinary Digital Engagement in Arts & Humanities*. Some small sections in Chapter 4 are accepted for publication as a chapter in the forthcoming book *EnTwine: A Critical and Creative Companion to Teaching with Twine* edited by Anastasia Salter and Stuart Moulthrop for Amherst College Press, 2024. A portion of Chapter 1, within the heading "Soul Cyster Dot Net," was published in a 2020 solo-authored article called "Illness of the Gendered Body, Freud's *The Uncanny*, and 'Being-in-the-World'" in the *Canadian Review of Comparative Literature*.

# 1 Introduction

*Sixty-three. That's the number of hairs that shed from my scalp today. I know this because I laid them out in a meticulous line to count. Being diagnosed with hyperandrogenism at 19 triggered a decade of obsessive compulsions: rituals of counting, picking, checking. Hyperandrogenism, a condition of "excessive" levels of testosterone in the female body, can cause "masculinizing" symptoms*[1] *including excess body and facial hair, male-pattern baldness, infertility, increased muscle mass and absence of menstrual bleeding (Bazarganipour et al. 371). Individuals with hyperandrogenism, I've learned, experience subjugation both culturally through the reinforcement of sex norms and institutionally through the pathologizing of deviant femininity. One night, whilst grappling with my newly formed sick*[2] *identity, I unearthed a blue-glowed haven: a digital health forum. Inside a message box, I began to write about my illness. My journey into the relatively unexplored field of digital illness narratives starts here…*

In *The Wounded Storyteller*, Arthur Frank wrote that major illness has the potential to disrupt the map that once guided our life. We have plans, aspirations, and goals when suddenly, in the wake of an unexpected diagnosis, we no longer can forge the path we once imagined because illness exposes the ableism in the lives we chart and narrate for ourselves. In the place of our former path, we become well acquainted with clinic waiting rooms, researching symptoms and prescription drug side effects. It is when we are claimed by a new *sick* identity that we are required to relinquish our narrative to the medical institution in ways that, Frank argues, reinforce the Cartesian dualism of a modern experience of being ill (6). In this modern experience, according to Frank, we are categorized in a binary of *sick* or *well*, and, through an objectifying process, our bodies become separate from our *selves* as we are required to share our narrative through the language of the institution. Scholars of illness narratives argue that it is through the practice of writing about one's experience of illness that the capacity for telling one's story is reclaimed (Frank 1). Illness narratives—autobiographical accounts of the experience of pathology or disability—can be particularly transformative for

DOI: 10.4324/9781003646921-1

marginalized groups as an accessible way to bring agency and voice to the body (Couser, *Signifying Bodies* 16).

Despite their therapeutic value, illness narratives are bound by limitations including barriers to entry for marginalized groups (Couser, *Signifying Bodies* 58). Life writing scholar G. Thomas Couser, for instance, recounts the evolution of life writing studies in his 2009 book *Signifying Bodies: Disability in Contemporary Life Writing*. Reflecting on his own academic journey, he recounts the mid-1970s when life writing primarily revolved around autobiography which held prominence due to its self-authorship and long-standing tradition in Western culture. The field of life writing studies, though, began to acknowledge its gender biases and the ways in which self-authorship forefronted certain voices over others. The criticisms extended to forms of illness-based life writing, drawing various questions within the field and the community: Who has access to traditional publishing practices? Whose life experiences are deemed narratable, and why? Why are certain illness experiences considered more worthy of publication than others? How can we turn to intersectional approaches to understanding capacity, labour, and the time required to sit and write a lengthy book? How do certain illnesses or disabilities affect capacity or inhibit the ability to sit and write a lengthy book? And crucially, how do we ensure that these stories, pushed to the margins, are heard as well?

Attention in scholarship then shifted to forms more inclusive of women and marginalized groups, such as letters, diaries, testimonies and relational narratives focusing on others close to the writer (Couser, *Signifying Bodies* 12). The term life writing emerged as an encompassing label for various practices devoted to portraying real individuals' lives, not necessarily confined to literary discourse. Couser notes how the digital age pulled in new postprint representations, like blogs and online diaries, allowing life writers to bypass traditional publishing gatekeepers. Online life writing, which began to emerge as a method of self-publishing, Couser argues, offers direct accessibility for individuals seeking to tell their stories but who lack access to traditional forms of publishing. Courser names this shift as a "democratization of life writing" (12).

I want to set traditional illness narrative aside for a moment and pull into focus a different narrative practice: literary hypertext. Literary hypertext is a form of digital story writing that calls on the reader to participate in the narrative's unfolding by selecting hyperlink options which branch the narrative into nonlinear directions. The past two decades has seen a strong revival of scholarly and public interest in the genre of literary hypertext, stemming from the access it allows marginalized game developers who are often excluded from masculinist, white spaces of game development (Anthropy 21). While there appears to be a method in the latter medium for addressing access barriers present in the former practice, there is limited scholarly research on the potential for literary hypertext as a tool for writing therapeutic illness narratives. This book explores how literary hypertext technology may be a valuable therapeutic method for writing illness narratives by turning to a distinct case study: women and nonbinary individuals with hyperandrogenism. This book argues that the therapeutic value of writing a literary hypertext illness narrative ultimately lies in the distinct process of mapping and charting reflective experiences through hyperlinks accompanied by sharing the narrative with the broader community. To truly cultivate meaningful therapeutic benefits, narratives should allow both the author and the wider social and medical community to reflect on and understand the subjective experience of illness.

In the corners of public discourse there exists a budding notion in regards to hyperandrogenism. It speaks of a perceived inadequacy within the normative healthcare system[3] in addressing the complex needs of individuals diagnosed with sex-based illness that incarnate nuances of biological sex embodiment.[4] Due to experiences of dismissal, a transactional relation or needs generally going unmet within the patient–physician encounter, patients are seeking community and support in alternative avenues, both within their local communities and in the online space. Despite the widespread prevalence of hyperandrogenism and the reported psychological distress experienced by those affected, particularly women (Karjula et al. 1861–1869), normative healthcare systems have demonstrated a lack of accountable, ethical and adequate care. Simultaneously, playing out on the public stage are media representations of "sex verification testing" narratives in Olympic contexts, as will be discussed in Chapter 4 of this book. Here, we see individuals with hyperandrogenism are colliding with both the systemic marginalization through cultural discourse and the pathologization of their identities in the medical encounter. Lacking sufficient guidance from medical professionals, some women diagnosed with hyperandrogenism have found refuge in online health forums where they are exchanging personal narratives of their lived experiences. But these spaces are not a holistic solution, and come with risks of their own. There is a deep and critical need for concrete, novel pathways, in the digital space, in private rooms, and inside, outside and alongside the normative healthcare system, to inform therapeutic approaches for emotional well-being related to sex-based illness. Literary hypertext is one promising, accessible method that can be taken up by individuals and clinicians to offer meaningful benefits, not only for individualized therapy, but for supporting broader social change through education.

The problem at the centre of this book is ultimately two-fold. First, as will be outlined in depth in Chapter 2, individuals with hyperandrogenism experience subjugation both culturally through the reinforcement of sex norms and institutionally through the pathologizing of deviant femininity. Due to this subjugation, some women and nonbinary individuals with hyperandrogenism are turning to the writing of illness narratives to grapple with their experiences. Therefore, the second problem this book responds to understands that despite the therapeutic value of traditional illness narratives, the genre has been challenged for upholding barriers to entry for marginalized groups (Couser, *Signifying Bodies* 58). In a distinct vein, the past two decades has seen a strong revival of scholarly and public interest in the genre of literary hypertext, stemming from the access it allows marginalized game developers who are often excluded from masculinist, white spaces of game development (Anthropy 21). However, there is limited research on the potential for literary hypertext as a tool for writing therapeutic illness narratives. This dualized problem then leads to the intention of this book which is to understand how literary hypertext technology may be a valuable therapeutic tool for writing illness narratives for women and nonbinary individuals with hyperandrogenism.

At the core of this project is the question: how can women and nonbinary individuals with hyperandrogenism use literary hypertext technology to write illness narratives that construct positive relationships between their identities and the world? The structure of this question is intentionally expansive and invites us to interpret the data in ways that identify both technical aspects of digital tools and thematic patterns in story worlds that may contribute to the development of positive relationship building for the hypertext author. In this sense, this question seeks to analyse both digital features of literary hypertext, as well as themes or insights about the experience of hyperandrogenism that emerge through literary hypertext illness narratives. Further, in asking this first foundational question, more questions emerge: how can hypertext be utilized to hone in on the transformative, therapeutic aspects of the illness narrative? How might these tools offer an effective and purposeful means for subjugated bodies to write a path to health liberation?[5] What is innovative or inventive about digital capability that advances the potential of illness narratives? This book considers how we might "code" health liberation into the digital for women and nonbinary people with hyperandrogenism through literary hypertext technology.

My intention is for this book to be one resource among many, offering a pathway forward for those feeling constrained by their *sick* identity. Perhaps you are grappling with a recent diagnosis of hyperandrogenism, or you may be a clinician seeking innovative approaches to therapeutic benefits for patients with sex-based illness. In either case, my hope is for this book to serve as a valuable resource, offering insights into the theoretical intersections of pathologized identities, literary hypertext, and illness narratives, along with a DIY guide to help you construct your own political narrative therapy-informed hypertext module, whether for personal use or to support a patient in need.

## Soul Cysters Dot Net

In March of 2015, a post entitled "Breaking Down Emotionally Over PCOS" was uploaded to the online health forum SoulCysters.net by an author using the handle htr12. The opening lines of the post read: "So I just found this site today, and i was diagnosed on October 31, 2008. I sort of gave up looking up info on PCOS for a month or so, because I just felt so hopless [sic]" (htr12). htr12 proceeds to tell their story of living with an endocrine disorder known as polycystic ovary syndrome (PCOS). The author's adolescence was plagued with irregular menstrual cycles, as little as two to four periods a year that they tried and failed to regulate with various brands of combined oral contraceptive pills. At the age of 18, htr12 recalls feeling distraught over the possibility that they might not be able to conceive in the future. This threat to future motherhood compelled the author to seek medical attention. They were advised by various physicians to continue alternative contraceptive pills in order to find the "right one," despite jumping between not menstruating for over eight months to constant spotting. htr12 notes that "3 of the docs made me feel like i was crazy, and told me to just keep taking the pills [sic]." The author describes a deep yearning for motherhood becoming more urgent as they began planning their wedding.

htr12 decided to attempt a physician visit again despite their past negative experiences. They write:

> I made another appointment 3 months later and the doc. gave me a preg test (which was neg) and told me that since i was not married that she should not be having this conversation with me about my period irregularities. I went home in tears and never wanted to go back to a doc again [sic]. (htr12)

Sometime later, the author eventually received a diagnosis of PCOS, an endocrine disorder which commonly causes infertility, among other symptoms. htr12 describes their emotional turmoil over the diagnosis and a potential inability to conceive as devastating. The author also describes how the experience isolates them from other women in their life because the author feels they cannot relate to the "ordinary" experience of womanhood. The author notes that some days are consumed with mourning over their "defective" body. The author describes their most recent emotional "breakdown," triggered by their cousin's "unplanned" pregnancy. The author recalls, "I was so jealous of them, and didn't even want to go near them… The few people i've told tell me they know how i feel, and they've had their children. No, you don't know how i feel, and i can't just get over it [sic]" (htr12). The author's post signs off with an extension of gratitude for the Soul Cysters message board where they believe they can discuss experiences with other women who understand their situation.

While many posts uploaded to Soul Cysters are open to view by anyone with an internet connection, testimonials such as htr12's offer a glimpse into what feels akin to a private support group, sitting within a circle of chairs amongst individuals navigating their identities in light of a PCOS diagnosis. PCOS is the most common metabolic and endocrine disorder for women of reproductive age, affecting from 6% to 26% of women (Lauritsen et al.). PCOS presents through a complex set of symptoms, including irregular menstrual cycles, infertility, insulin resistance, weight gain and polycystic ovaries, however, it is hyperandrogenism that particularly captures my attention. Hyperandrogenism is a complex condition because it may occur alongside several underlying conditions of DSD or endocrine disorders including PCOS, Congenital Adrenal Hyperplasia, Cushing's syndrome, among others (Rachoń 205). Hyperandrogenism is a fascinating condition because it destabilizes certain, established belief systems surrounding biological sex, ones deeply ingrained in our cultural fabric. These beliefs have seeped into our institutions, from healthcare to the Olympics, and work to shape our understanding of gender and health. Yet, as we grapple with the implications of hyperandrogenism, a fundamental question emerges: What does it mean to be *sick*? It is a question that I have thought a lot about in the past ten years and it has challenged me to reconsider the very essence of *sickness* and its intersections with identity.

htr12's testimonial, and others like it that populate the Soul Cysters forum, collectively pull towards a common concern that medical institutions are failing to provide effective and meaningful support for PCOS (Sterling et al. S7), compelling these women to seek alternative communities both physical and in the online space. Despite the disorder's prevalence, and the documented suffering and distress reported by women with PCOS (Karjula et al. 1861–1869), the medical system has failed to provide accountable, ethical and responsible support for women with PCOS (Sterling et al. S7), including htr12. Unsupported by a medical system, some women diagnosed with PCOS have turned to online health forums as a place in which to share testimonials based on their lived experience. I was one of those women.

I was 15 when I found myself grappling with, what I perceived as, a second puberty. These bodily changes, unlike the shared experiences of adolescence where our secondary sex characteristics typically morph in tandem with our peers, I found myself confronting these later changes alone. I first started to notice the acne, then the excessive body hair, and, finally, the hair loss on my scalp. It contributed to an anxiety disorder and, later, a diagnosis of obsessive compulsive disorder. I became consumed with body-focused thoughts and this compulsion to constantly check body parts for new, abrupt changes. Reflecting on those early adult years, there is a single image my mind comes back to: the clinic waiting room. Countless hours of my life were spent sitting in a plastic chair waiting for the receptionist to call my name and invite me into a consultation with a series of clinicians—general practitioners, naturopathic doctors, acupuncturists, nutritionists, dermatologists, endocrinologists and obstetrician–gynaecologists. Every visit followed a formula: recounting the story of my body—its abnormality, its unpredictability—and receiving a prescription or advice from the clinician in return. I cycled through a suite of medications which offered temporary relief. They would mostly slow the onslaught of unwanted hair growth or clear up my acne, but, in time I was always met with side effects. It became a cycle of addressing symptoms with more medications. I had to buy a custom, oversized pill organizer just to manage it all.

It was during this time that I turned to the digital space. I typed "PCOS Help" into the search bar so often it became my first autofill result. As I remember this time, I scraped the internet barrels of every site that mentioned my condition. The 11th or 12th search result was SoulCyster.net. Here, for the first time, I found something that was new in my experience of illness: shared experiences of women who were coming to terms with the same issues as I was. I failed to realize until then just how isolating illness could be. Now, it was notable because for the first time I was hearing the experiences of others. I know now that I was stepping into a global sisterhood where stories of success and loss with PCOS were exchanged freely, strategies for navigating doctor's appointments and managing side effects were dissected with empathy and understanding, and, critically, women were diagnosing each other. More on that to come.

I was searching for a topic for my master's thesis a few years later and I found myself returning to the exploration of feminist community building in the online space. I had just taken a course on the history of feminist print production, which led me to think about the legacy of feminist print as a tool for consciousness-raising. This pulled me down a research path exploring feminist community formation and how it manifests in our digital world. A faculty member in my department at the time advised me to "write what you know" and it struck me that sickness was something I knew very intimately. I decided, then, to focus my thesis on how some women are turning to online illness narratives to write their "abject" bodies (Butler, *Bodies that Matter* 3) into a budding corporeal politic. My research examined the writing in SoulCysters.net as illness narrative and explored the types of discourses on gender and illness that were developing in this online space.

When I began conceptualizing my master's research, I imagined that Soul Cysters was wholly a site of resistance to normative ways of responding to illness, particularly through the healthcare system. However, I found that multiple, deviating dialogues were emerging: women were expressing empowerment and support in community, yet, at the same time, (re)producing discursive hegemonic femininity (Perram 2017; Schippers 85). Both the normative medical system and the Soul Cysters community were mandating a standard of femininity for women with PCOS. In the same way, healthcare policies enable physicians to prescribe medications and perform procedures that combat "masculine" bodily expressions, the Soul Cysters community reinforced these same objectives. Physicians look to treat the bodies of women with PCOS through prescribing androgen blocker medications such as Spironolactone, oral and topical Minoxidil for male-pattern baldness, hair removal procedures such as laser and electrolysis, or hair growth prevention cream like Vaniqa (Lucidi). Much of the discourse on Soul Cysters reaffirmed the pursuit to access these prescriptions, or at least the results the prescriptions promise.

Despite the community of the Soul Cysters forum working in transgressive ways which re-centre the subjectivity of these women, I found that the objective of discussions in this space was to discover new ways to attain normative femininity. Women in the Soul Cysters blog share alternative treatments used to lower androgen excess, to re-grow hair on their heads and diminish the hair on their bodies. These women share collective pain and mourning over their inability to become pregnant without a collective resistance to essentialist notions which inherently link womanhood to motherhood. The Soul Cysters rehearse scripts to perform to physicians so that they may receive the diagnoses and accompanying prescriptions they want. This subversion, however, is ultimately to obtain more efficient and accessible ways to combat the perceived masculinization of their bodies.

This is where we pause to bring home the critical facet of this finding. This is not to say that regulating gender is not imperative to the livelihoods of women and individuals with PCOS and hyperandrogenism, because it is. Nor is it to undermine the severe injustice women with PCOS face in the healthcare system or the lack of funding or mobilization PCOS draws for medical research. As the structures of oppression currently stand, these injustices for women with PCOS mean discrimination, alienation and punishment of their bodily expressions insofar as they destabilize our societal understandings of gender. As I came to understand that the Soul Cysters blog replicates the gender regulations of the healthcare system and beyond, I also came to understand why. As Judith Butler argues, achieving gender normalcy is an effort of survival (*Undoing Gender* 100).

Ultimately, our practices for reading a sexed body are socially constituted, but this does not mean that gender, as a "mode of becoming,"[6] is trivial

(Butler, *Undoing Gender* 217). Gender affects us in deeply meaningful ways and there are serious implications when the sexed body is read "incorrectly" or when it is unreadable at all. These implications include both social persecution where performing gender "appropriately" becomes a mode of survival, and internal disarray when one's process of becoming is stifled or halted. It is understandable, then, why the Soul Cysters reproduce standard femininity. Meeting this standard becomes either a process of survival or a mode of becoming. For the Soul Cysters, the online community becomes meaningful in their process of becoming, and how that process intersects with their *sick* identity. Critically, this online space was providing them something valuable that they were not finding in the normative health care system. From here, I began to wonder how that "something" could be harnessed.

## *Click Me*: The Research Project

When I began work on my dissertation, I was eager to continue exploring hyperandrogenism illness narratives, albeit through a different methodological lens. At that time, I was completing a research assistantship for a project called *Writing New Bodies* (Ensslin et al. *Writing New Bodies*). In *Writing New Bodies* we turned to feminist participatory action research and critical community co-design to craft an interactive digital story app, known in some spaces as digital fiction. Our aim was to provide a medium for media-enhanced bibliotherapy—or reading as a form of therapy—to help young women and nonbinary individuals from diverse backgrounds in building resilience against body image concerns.

One of my responsibilities in my research assistantship role involved designing and facilitating workshops for young women and nonbinary participants across Canada. Within these workshops, we utilized literary hypertext software, empowering participants to build the stories of their bodies in creative ways. We had participants respond to various body-based writing prompts by constructing personal stories using literary hypertext software. Some workshops involved collaborative narrative building, while others encouraged solitary writing sessions accompanied by music, with sharing at the end for those who were interested. Witnessing the overwhelmingly positive response to this aspect of the workshops was truly remarkable. Many participants expressed how the software's accessibility and the opportunity to set free their creativity through storytelling made it the most impactful part of the weekend they spent with us. This experience triggered the initial connection for me between literary hypertext as a method to revolutionize illness narratives.

In March 2020, I began working closely with a group of women and nonbinary participants who self-identify[7] as having hyperandrogenism in my dissertation research, which, at the time, was called "Click Me: Literary Hypertext as Illness Narrative for Women and Nonbinary Individuals with Hyperandrogenism." As discussed above, hyperandrogenism is an endocrine condition characterized by "excessive" levels of male hormones (androgens), such as testosterone which, when identified in the female body, are associated with "masculinizing" symptoms including excess body and facial hair, male-pattern baldness, infertility, elevated sex drive, increased muscle mass and absence of menstrual bleeding (Bazarganipour et al. 371). The participants I worked with were English speakers who are at least 18 years old and have at least two clinical symptoms of hyperandrogenism. I recruited participants from Facebook support groups for PCOS,[8] Instagram, email listservs and public online health forums. Informed by my experience supporting the related research design of *Writing New Bodies*, I recruited ten participants as this size is expansive representationally but narrow enough for focused engagement. The recruitment method was intentional in order to connect with individuals who may have been seeking support or information on their disease, digitally.

Following screening and consent seeking processes, participants were sent a link to a two-hour digital module that they could complete in a location where they felt most comfortable, and at their own pace. The module was designed using Twine,[9] a freely accessible, open-source tool for creating literary hypertexts. The module was intentionally designed through the lens of political narrative therapy, drawing from the work of Renee Dumaresque, Taylor Thornton, Daniela Glaser and Anthony Lawrence in their article "Politicized Narrative Therapy." This approach integrates anti-colonial discursive frameworks, critical race theory, counter-storytelling, Black feminist thought and anti-sanist theorizing to re-conceptualize narrative therapy as a catalyst for political transformation. Dumaresque et al.'s political narrative therapy framework was effective for this project because it is able to walk in tandem with Martinez and Fleck-Henderson's concept of health liberation, as noted earlier in this chapter. Embracing health liberation, and particularly political narrative therapy, reframes illness as a societal injustice rather than a purely individual affliction, advocating for solutions rooted in social, institutional and political realms.

The Twine module includes information on, and a political framing of, hyperandrogenism, a story-boarding exercise, a Twine software tutorial, and a final writing prompt that participants used to build their own literary hypertext stories rooted in their illness experiences. When participants completed their illness narratives, they uploaded them to a personalized, secure folder. From there, I invited the participant to a closing interview to discuss their experience using literary hypertext to write an illness narrative and to reflect on what kind of changes, if any, they experienced after writing. This completed the participants' involvement in the study. Following the closing interview, participants were invited to submit their Twine stories to a private, secure online space to which only myself and the other participants had access. It was explained to participants that this portal would act as a community-building space where participants could read each other's illness stories. Participants were informed that submitting their story to this space was optional, did not affect their participation in the study (if they chose not to share, I would still use their data), and that their submission would remain anonymous. All ten participants chose to share their stories. These stories have become the foundation of this book and are explored in depth in later chapters. Throughout this book, when I refer to this project, I will call the illness narrative module the *Click Me* module and I will refer to the participants as the *Click Me* authors.

## A Note on Language

When you are working on a project that looks at embodied experience that is typically pathologized as a medical condition that interferes with normative ways of understanding biological sex, categories of defining gender and illness become muddy. In this book, I require a term to define the *Click Me* authors. Clinical guidelines in North America for defining people with hyperandrogenism use the term *woman* (Yildiz 167), however, it became apparent that this term is gravely insufficient to describe all individuals who experience the condition. Hyperandrogenism, a condition diagnosed in "female" bodies that produce "excess" male hormones is complex because it diagnostically relies on binary language that does not reflect the population of people who experience it. For example, I have a nonbinary author who took part in this study who self-identifies as having hyperandrogenism. From here it may logically lead to a conclusion that the phrase I should use to define my population would be *women and nonbinary people*. This is the phrase I do employ in this book and it does, in fact, define my population of ten authors. However, this phrase does not represent all individuals who identify as having hyperandrogenism. A transgender man may, for example, have extensive experience, even in the healthcare system, with hyperandrogenism. From here, it may appear using the phrase *assigned female at birth* could represent the population of individuals who identify as having hyperandrogenism. Though, I began to wonder if this is universally true.

Hyperandrogenism is closely tied to, and even in some contexts (mis) understood as, a diagnosis of "intersex" or DSD (Davis and Preves 80).[10] It is plausible that an individual who identifies as having hyperandrogenism may not have been assigned female at birth and may, in fact, have been assigned differently (male, or in some jurisdictions a "third" sex classifier). This fact leads to the obvious solution that I should refer to the population in a general way, such as *individuals* or *people* (terms which I do employ at times). However, the glaring issue with this solution is that it works to erase the very gendered implications of the disease of hyperandrogenism. The issues of hyperandrogenism that this project explores are the ways in which, medically and culturally, the disease is viewed as a condition that masculinizes the "female" body.

Many of the issues that individuals with hyperandrogenism face, including many of the *Click Me* authors, are issues around perceptions of not being able to embody an idea of femininity and the kinds of psychological impacts that may have. Further, the condition raises issues for individuals around the ways in which their gender is read, or misread, in society (see Fausto-Sterling; Stryker and Whittle). At the same time, nonbinary people and transgender men's relationship to the illness may be different from femme-identifying people. A lot of the distress surrounding hyperandrogenism is around the "masculinizing symptoms" and these symptoms may or may not induce similar distress in transgender men or nonbinary people. However, for the *Click Me* authors, anxiety around not meeting a standard of femininity was a central theme.

Because of this reality, and what I would argue is the most significant aspect of hyperandrogenism for this book, it is imperative for me to maintain language around constructed femininity and womanhood. However, I want to do this by also including those who may not identify with these terms directly. The solution I have chosen is three-fold. First, I will refer to the *Click Me* authors by the gender terms they have identified within screening interviews: *women* and *nonbinary people*. Second, I will refer to the larger population as *individuals* with hyperandrogenism, as this is the only terminology that captures all identities. Third, the exclusionary phrase *women with hyperandrogenism* will only be used when referring directly to the language of others whom I am discussing (e.g., diagnostic language or language a *Click Me* author includes in their story).

The label of pathologized illness has historically and is contemporarily used to categorize what some emerging identity communities would now call *differing embodiments*, *ways of being* or *identity categories* (nuances of biological sex embodiments, fat bodies, disability, madness, etc.) (Kelly and Orsini 288; Svenaeus, "The Body Uncanny" 125; Sulik 463). Pathologized identities are complex. Some individuals or communities may view *a way of being* as an illness in the traditional sense and others may find the label reductive or subjugating. Further, these same communities or individuals who may find these labels harmful in some sense (it defines their embodiments as abnormal, for example) may seek pathologized labels for the resources they can afford (particular healthcare procedures, medications, insurance coverage, etc.). For those who embrace illness labels for their embodiments, this too can be a liberatory act. Defining oneself as ill may be a step towards validation of experience and following a treatment path within the normative healthcare system may be extremely beneficial for some.

This book will use the term *pathologized identity* (with a cheeky *sick* identity littered throughout), to describe individuals with hyperandrogenism and the term *illness* to refer to the condition of hyperandrogenism, for three reasons. First, these terms speak to difference as an identity category, however, they do not erase the ways in which these *ways of being* are pulled into diagnostic criteria of illness, or are descriptors of the illness themselves. Second, *pathologized* as a verb form works to represent how some people's bodies are pulled into a discourse of pathology with or without their consent or desire. Some pathologized identities experience the act of the pathologizing of their identity and this act is without a value judgment. Third, *pathologized identities* allows for a thematic connection to illness narratives as a responsive action. The history of the practice of illness narratives is rooted in a desire to push back against the perceived omnipotence of the healthcare system and reposition illness as a sociohistorical experience rather than merely a bodily state (see Couser; Frank; Hawkins; Kleinman). However, the term *illness* in *illness narratives* is retained. Perhaps *illness* can be seen as both a restrictive and generative label. Like *illness, pathologized identity* is fluid as there is no set of experiences or embodiments that always occupy the category for everyone, but the term can be used as a tool to think more critically about the processes of diagnosing and treating illness as historically situated and sociopolitically constituted.

## Illness Narratives

Illness narrative is a relatively new genre that has migrated to the forefront of scholarly interest in the past thirty years, taken up in the fields of medicine, sociology, psychology, ethics and later, medical/health humanities, narrative medicine and narrative therapy. The emergence of illness narratives as a scholarly discipline can be understood as two-fold. The early development of the genre can be traced to an exploration of the role of personal narratives in medicine and healthcare (as will be discussed below through the works of scholars Arthur Kleinman, Anne Hunsaker Hawkins, Rita Charon and Craig Irvine). In this context, illness narrative is emerging as a subset of narrative medicine within the wider discipline of medicine. At the same time, literary scholars and cultural theorists were also beginning to explore the ways in which personal narratives about illness and disability could challenge dominant cultural narratives about health and the body (as will be discussed below in the narratives of Martha Weinman Lear and Norman Cousin).

In this second context, illness narrative is emerging as a genre of literature that goes on to intersect with development in gender and disability studies. Here is where the distinct discipline of health/medical humanities emerges as an interdisciplinary field of study that explores the intersection of medicine, healthcare and the humanities. Health/medical humanities pulls in perspectives and theories, as well as scholars and practitioners, from a collection of disciplines, including literature, philosophy, history, anthropology, art and ethics. Ultimately, the discipline expands understanding of health and illness beyond purely biological factors to include social, cultural and political implications. We can see that the medical and literary roots of the illness narrative genre collide to produce some aspects of health/medical humanities as shown through the more contemporary work of illness narrative scholars Arthur Frank, G. Thomas Couser and Stella Bolaki. Today, illness narratives is an expansive field of inquiry that turns to a broad range of artefacts from historical diaries to virtual reality (VR) games to literary hypertext.

One of the introductory moments of the conceptualization of illness narratives as a scholarly genre was the publication of the momentous 1988 book, *The Illness Narratives: Suffering, Healing, and the Human Condition* by the medical anthropologist and psychiatrist, Arthur Kleinman. Kleinman became a leading proponent of the perspective that illness holds social meaning for those who are affected and that this meaning should be analyzed and understood by the discipline of medicine. Five years later, Anne Hunsaker Hawkins wrote the innovative *Reconstructing Illness: Studies in Pathography*, the first account of the term pathography to describe the genre of illness narratives. Hawkins was a pioneer in the development of the nursing informatics field, which looks at the use of information technology and data analysis in the practice of nursing. Hawkins' use of the term pathography was to describe a subgenre of autobiography that centres personal accounts of illness (3). Hawkins explains that the novel scholarship on pathography is a response to a lack of documented illness narratives as a historically popular genre.

Before 1950, it was uncommon for publishers to support book projects that detailed nonfictional experiences of illness, and before the 1900s this genre was seemingly absent (Hawkins 3). As Hawkins describes, attempting to classify published pathographies was complex as most cataloguing systems at that time organized works based on disease type. These methods, though, work to centre the illness over the author's experience, an outcome that the pathography genre tends to oppose. Therefore, Hawkins moves to classify pathographies by author intent which filters work into three defining categories: testimonial pathographies, angry pathographies and pathographies advocating alternative modes of treatment (4).

In the 1960s and 1970s, testimonial pathographies were characterized by stark religious overtones and explicitly worked to reinforce spiritual faith, affirm the authority of formal medicine and maintain an optimistic tone to provide solace to readers navigating similar health challenges. By the 1980s, pathographies of anger emerged which collectively articulated contempt for the healthcare system, while simultaneously, spoke of dualized suffering—both from the illness itself and from depersonalized medical encounters. A seminal example is Martha Weinman Lear's *Heartsounds* (1980), which exposes systemic medical negligence and the resultant victimization of patients. The third category, which advocates for alternative modes of treatment, surfaced in the late 1970s with Norman Cousin's *Anatomy of an Illness*. While similarly critical of conventional medical practices, these narratives emphasize the exploration of holistic and alternative healing methodologies and ultimately reject Cartesian dualism in favour of an integrated mind–body paradigm. This shift towards self-authority in health and the reconceptualization of the mind–body relationship has significantly influenced contemporary illness narrative scholarship, as shown in the works of Arthur Frank, Craig Irvine, Rita Charon and G. Thomas Couser.

One of the more accessible scholarly accounts of illness narratives came in 1995 with the publication of Frank's book on narrative theory entitled *The Wounded Storyteller*. Frank, a leader in the field of medical sociology and narrative medicine, explores the notion of the "remission society" where mass communities ritualistically weave in and out of the *sick* identity label leaving them "well but not cured" (8). Frank draws on illness accounts from authors such as Oliver Sacks, Anatole Broyard, Norman Cousins and Audre Lorde to outline three main arguments. First, Frank expresses a need for the ill to reclaim their life stories, arguing that this reclamation is an act of forging new paths of agency for those who have been subjugated by their experiences. Second, Frank makes a stark condemnation of the Cartesian mind–body split to which Western healthcare seemingly subscribes (1). Instead, Frank argues for the patient's embodiment of their illness narrative, as these stories are "told not just about the body but through it" (3).

His rejection of Cartesian dualism is reinforced by his third topic which explores the evolution of the body in relation to medicine from pre-modern to postmodern times. Frank maps the dominant experience of illness beginning at premodernity through modernity to postmodernity arguing that this evolution shows an expansion of the significance of the patient's voice (7). In the realm of premodernity, the *sick* would "go to bed and die, cared for by family members and neighbours with talent for healing" (Frank 5). In the transition to modernity, medical terminology and knowledge were gatekept by medical professionals who required the patient to forfeit not only their bodies but also their life narratives to the medical institution. But there was also an influx of technological expertise, complex diagnostics and medical progress through pharmacology and other treatments. Frank argues that this new experience of hope in relation to healing was perplexing for a society that understood illness as a mystery. Modernity brought recovery at the expense of chronic illness, relapse and "watch-and-wait" advice (where serious illness is identified in the early stages where no treatment is available until it progresses).

Frank argues that modernity became a network of storytelling where patients share their narratives of experience with medical professionals who, in turn, translate those stories into data. Once this data is filtered through the medical pathways, the patient's reinterpreted narrative of the body is told back to them. However, the story no longer belongs to the patient but to the medical institution that claims their retelling as empirical truth. Frank argues that the experience of illness in the time of modernity involves the active colonization of the patient's body by the medical institution which ultimately views the mind as distinct from the experience of the body. The *sick* body in modernity is an empty vessel that becomes objectified in the illness experience rather than viewed as inseparable from the patient's sense of self. Postmodernity, for Frank, is a "postcolonial demand for voice" by the patient (13). Here, the illness becomes a reclaiming of agency where patients begin to observe that there is more meaning in the experience of illness outside the narrative capacity of the medical institution. Ultimately, postmodernity for Frank is "when the capacity for telling one's story is reclaimed" (7).

Frank understands elements of illness narratives as classifiable and defined by one of three narrative typologies: restitution, quest or chaos. Each narrative typology, for Frank, describes a different experience of being ill and illness narratives can incorporate multiple typologies. Unlike Hawkins' classifying system which seemingly uses a thematic categorization, Frank turns to the lived experience of the author. Restitution narratives centre around a collective goal of achieving health again. The role of those who encounter the patient, such as physicians, healthcare workers and family, are like-minded agents of the patient's recovery. Frank argues, that in his own experience of illness, retribution narratives felt like a stripping of his agency. This typology tends to position the physician as the heroic protagonist in a narrative where the patient becomes the object to manipulate whose wily nature must be conquered (XIV). Chaos narratives, according to Frank, explore the unravelling of self that accompanies many experiences of illness. Chaos narratives sift through the complexities of diagnostic uncertainty when a patient's experience of pain or discomfort cannot be readily identified by the healthcare system (XIV). Chaos subsides once validation of experience is achieved by the patient, which may look like a diagnosis or recognition of pain and suffering. Finally, illness as quest emerges for Frank through narrative moments that work to resist sentiments of a diminished life, a feeling that tends to accompany the progression of a fatal disease. Quest narratives value the significance and meaning of a life in its entirety rather than a snapshot at its ending.

Following Frank's prolific work came an influx of scholarly inquiry into the illness narrative genre, particularly in the fields of medical/health humanities and narrative medicine in relation to ethics. In 1997, G. Thomas Couser wrote *Recovering Bodies: Illness Disability and Life Writing* which, for the field of illness narratives, has become a foundational work that intersects disability studies and autobiography. Couser has become known for his contributions to the field of disability studies and for his work on the intersections of literature, culture and disability. In *Recovering Bodies*, Couser profiles the writing of individuals with disability or illness, including individuals with HIV/AIDS, breast cancer, deafness and paralysis, and argues for both the resisting of stigma and the reclamation of the body from medicalized discourse through the telling of one's story.

Couser went on to contribute to the foundations of illness narrative scholarship through his authoring of *Vulnerable Subjects: Ethics and Life Writing* (2004) and *Signifying Bodies: Disability in Contemporary Life Writing* (2009). In Couser's publication of *Signifying Bodies*, he continues his inquiry into the relationship between disability and narrative identity. Emerging at the heels of a legacy of institutionalized ableism that questions what a life worthy of living looks like, Couser turns to the autobiographical accounts of those living with disabilities. Couser argues that narratives of disability either reinforce or push back against "preferred rhetorics" of narrative. These preferred rhetorics typically see a normative trajectory of plot that may fall into one of several categories: triumphalist, gothic, spiritual compensation and nostalgic. Triumph narratives of disability work to deny impairment by insisting on "overcoming" the confines of a "defective body" as seen through common stories of blind runners or deaf musicians, for example (Couser, *Signifying Bodies* 33). Couser notes that this

> paradigm holds up the Supercrip, who is by definition atypical, as the model disabled person. These may be 'true stories,' but they are not truly representative lives. In any case this approach removes the stigma of disability from the author but leaves it in place for other individuals with the condition in question.
>
> (Couser, *Signifying Bodies* 33–34)

Another common disability narrative that works to reinforce hegemonic discourse, according to Couser, is horror or gothic narratives that explore themes of disfigurement, dreadful conditions and shunning of the protagonist from their community (*Signifying Bodies* 33). Gothic narratives of disability work to evoke a sense of either pity or the prejudicial revulsion of the author. Narratives of spiritual compensation work through sentiments of "God's plan" where stories typically begin with a "symbolic paradigm of disability, according to which an impairment is a mark of sin or God's displeasure with an individual" (Couser, *Signifying Bodies* 36). Through a series of obstacles that have been overcome by the author, eventually, they come to believe that their disability is in fact a gift from God granting them either a mission or a higher purpose for their life. Finally, narratives of nostalgia evoke a yearning for the past before disability in order to grapple with a loss of hope in being able to return to this reality (Couser, *Signifying Bodies* 39). Each of these four hegemonic paradigms of disability narratives actively work, according to Couser, to both maintain and create a system of oppression against those living with disabilities. This is because narratives of triumph, horror, spiritual compensation and nostalgia always return to the disabled body as abject.

In response to hegemonic narratives of disability, Couser argues, there has emerged a novel category of a counterhegemonic and postcolonial challenging narrative style: the rhetoric of emancipation. This counterhegemonic narrative style is upheld by the pillars of subversion, self-creation, self-possession and self-assertion. Most significantly, these narratives are inherently political in nature. The rhetoric of emancipation is attuned to the political struggle of identity for disabled people and ultimately calls for institutional recognition of the humanity and rights of those with disabilities (Couser, *Signifying Bodies* 47). Couser turns to the example of the 1989 autobiography *I Raise My Eyes to Say Yes* by Ruth Sienkiewicz-Mercer and Steven B. Kaplan. The book details the life story of Ruth, a woman born with a severe form of cerebral palsy that impacted her ability to move, speak and write. Ruth spent decades in rehabilitation centres and hospitals where physicians would routinely wrongfully assess her as lacking both intellectual and communicative capacity. In her story, Ruth discusses her discovery of communication through her gaze, and the new ways she was able to engage with the world after this breakthrough. However, Couser's description of narratives of triumph, Ruth's story "decisively represents disability not as a flaw in her body but as the prejudicial construct of a normative culture" (*Signifying Bodies* 47).

Ruth becomes political in a way that calls into inquiry the institutional treatment of disability and how it works to actively "other" the disabled experience. Further, Ruth's liberation is found not in approaching a state of "recovery" from her disability, but rather, from constituting her sense of identity in ways that challenge normative medicalized discourse. Couser observes that the woman's self-construction heavily relies on her own gaze. While the medical gaze initially labelled her as mentally deficient, her own inquisitive and assertive gaze allowed her to contest or reject this misdiagnosis and, importantly, to lead a social life. Once her intelligence and awareness were acknowledged, she further developed and refined her communication method, but she always maintained her assertive approach (Couser, *Signifying Bodies* 43). Ultimately, Ruth's narrative of emancipation advocates for the political paradigm of disability that seeks to subvert traditional medicine's pathologization of "abject" bodies. This framework of the rhetoric of emancipation is valuable for thinking about the pathologization of deviant femininity in relation to hyperandrogenism. Disability and hyperandrogenism parallel the experience of embodying the abject that ultimately must be "cured" in order to achieve a "healthy" state.

In 2004, Couser wrote *Vulnerable Subjects* which argues that illness narratives can be an accessible genre for vulnerable people to express themselves, however, there are a multitude of complexities when considering narrative agency in relation to illness (*Vulnerable Subjects* 14). Although illness narratives have the potential to be a liberating practice, traditional modes of publishing and writing narratives complicate consent. Certain illnesses or disabilities, Couser argues, can limit how a person is able to write or publish their story and this is where narrative partnerships may move to the forefront. Partnerships of publication, assisting authors, transcribers, translators and ghostwriters in relation to illness narratives must be attuned to a biomedical ethic to maintain the agency and voice of the author. Couser turns to the Four Principles of Biomedical Ethics originally developed by Thomas Beauchamp and James Childress in their 1979 book *Principles of Biomedical Ethics* which are currently utilized in modern bioethical decision-making: respect for autonomy, nonmaleficence, beneficence and justice. As Couser notes, these four principles

> seem pertinent to life writing, and all may come into play in different ways. (And as in bioethics, these principles represent only prima facie obligations; that is, they are binding only when no conflicting obligations override them. Thus, they are not absolute and inflexible).
>
> (*Vulnerable Subjects* 17)

With the emergence of the discipline of narrative medicine, as spearheaded by scholars such as Rita Charon and Craig Irvine, there has been a call to evaluate the shortcomings of biomedical principlism. Irvine and Charon argue in their 2017 chapter "Deliver Us from Certainty: Training for Narrative Ethics" in Charon et al.'s edited collection *The Principles and Practice of Narrative Medicine*, that reading the narratives of others offers a way into "envisioning otherness" (112). To envision otherness is to fortify a structure where readers can better understand the experiences of those who are marginalized through illness. However, as Irvine and Charon suggest, biomedical principlism argues that the oath to "do no harm" employed by physicians is, in fact, insufficient. This is because biomedical principlism insists on its universality when it has the potential to be interpreted differently by different physicians or pillars of medical discourse. The ability of physicians to contest and debate what they believe constitutes harm works to generate the illusion that they are omnipotent to the experiences and embodiment of the patient (Irvine and Charon 116).

Irvine and Charon, then, put the notion of casuistry forward as a foil to principlism. Casuistry is a method of ethical reasoning that focuses on the analysis of particular cases or situations to inform an application of general principles or rules. The authors argue that this approach centres the unique, individualized experiences of the patient rather than attempting to fit this experience into a prototype. The authors discuss the concept of narrative ethics, emphasizing the importance of understanding and addressing the unique life stories of patients in medical treatment. They argue that practicing narrative ethics involves exercising compassion by tailoring treatment to individual circumstances, rather than adhering rigidly to universal principles of justice. This approach requires narrative skill to effectively tend to each patient's specific needs and virtues, recognizing that ethical actions are context-dependent and manifest in unique situations with particular individuals (Irvine and Charon 120). Casuistry parallels Frank's notion of *shading* as the act of analyzing a narrative in both its contextual wholeness and uniqueness. Ultimately, Irvine and Charon argue, casuistry has become the foundation of narrative medicine today, which foregrounds a narrative ethic attuned to lived experience, nuance and feminist and structural justice frameworks (119).

In recent years, the trajectory of illness narrative scholarship has begun theorizing the proliferation of the genre in the digital space. In 2018, scholar Steve Rains wrote *Coping with Illness Digitally* which looks at the ways in which new media is being utilized to cope with illness, particularly responding to illness through the use of communication technologies like social media. Most notably, Rains reviews a series of studies that look at the potential of illness narratives online (see Anthony and Nagel; Graham et al.) and finds that engaging in this genre can be therapeutic and compared to more traditional forms of mental health therapy (69). Rains notes that illness blogging can be particularly beneficial as a therapeutic tool as it has been shown to be a generative agent where individuals can examine, reflect and engage with their life stories (69). According to Rains, blogging about life stress factors in relation to illness holds "cathartic potential" and "may serve to make one feel empowered, relieved, and even exhilarated" (69). Significantly, Rains also concludes that the therapeutic benefits of expressive writing about illness online were amplified by the ability to receive digital comments from others who have read their story (70). This is particularly valuable insight for the *Click Me* research because it speaks to the novel capabilities of online writing that cannot be fulfilled through traditional modalities of print publication. The uniqueness of the digital space allows for the cultivation of the online network and digital community that can engage with each other in real time through comment, chat or re-post functions.

According to the literature, illness narratives stand as a multifaceted practice for individuals to express and traverse their experiences with illness. For some who have endured institutionalized subjugation from the healthcare system and beyond, the practice of writing about one's illness subjectivity has served as a way to resist or undermine the authority of the medical establishment through self-representation (Couser, *Signifying Bodies* 31). Illness narrative, both as a research subject and as a personal practice, has a diversified, expansive scope. As Stella Bolaki, disability studies scholar and medical humanist, argues in her 2016 book *Illness as Many Narratives: Arts, Medicine and Culture*, approaches to illness narrative across time have been dynamic. Traditional perspectives have positioned the genre as a static, linear account of a relationship between biomedicine and the patient–physician encounter (Bolaki 1). This viewpoint benefits the authority of the medical establishment and fails to acknowledge illness narrative's history as a form of self-determination and resistance for marginalized identities (Couser, *Signifying Bodies* 31). Within the disciplines that engage with illness narrative, Bolaski calls for "critical interloping" which would invite interdisciplinary approaches to open up analysis for more nuanced research. This push for a more dynamic engagement with illness narrative recognizes the practice as manifold rather than one-dimensional and invites space for narrative complexities such as "formlessness" or "silence" (Bolaki 5). Bolaski exposes a new horizon for illness narratives beyond traditional practices of the linear written memoir to include the possibility of narrative multiplicity present in the digital space.

## Against Narrativity

Along with the swift influx of a scholarly embrace of narrative medicine came pushback. Authors, patients and scholars began challenging the sweeping claims of the discipline, assumptions around cultivating empathy for physicians, and the role of the patient as a storyteller. In 2004, Galen Strawson published "Against Narrativity" which challenges two identified pillars of narrative medicine scholarship: first, that people inherently understand their lives as a story and second, that this narrativizing of the self is a good thing (428). He argues that there exist individuals who are fundamentally non-narrative in their outlook and lifestyles. Ultimately, perspectives which disregard or devalue this non-narrative approach limit human self-awareness, restrict important avenues of thinking, diminish our understanding of ethical choices, cause unnecessary distress to those who deviate from narrative norms, and could be harmful in psychotherapeutic settings (Strawson 429). In his analysis, Strawson develops a conceptual framework for two opposing embodiments of the self: diachronic and episodic. The former, according to Strawson, tends to understand themselves as a temporal entity existing in the past and future, whereas the latter does not. This classification of the diachronic versus episodic sparked a series of scholarly reflections (see Battersby; Mackenzie and Poltera; Phelan; Schechtman; Tammi). Strawson began to open up space that is highly sceptical of strong claims made by narrative medicine and its proponents.

What followed was a series of works extending this scepticism. Frank, as the symbol of the wounded storyteller, became the focus of a number of these criticisms. Angela Woods, for example, published "Beyond the Wounded Storyteller: Rethinking Narrativity, Illness and Embodied Self-Experience" in the 2012 *Health, Illness and Disease: Philosophical Essays*. In this chapter,

Woods uses Strawson's arguments to challenge narrative medicine's perceived belief that we are all narrative selves and therefore the most optimal and healthy way to respond to illness is through the practice of narrative. Woods makes important critiques of Frank's classification of illness narrative genres, in particular. She argues that illness is inherently transformative, either leading to positive change, as seen in quest narratives, or negative outcomes, as depicted in chaos narratives. According to this perspective, stories of recovery are perceived as belonging to individuals in denial, disconnected from reality, or influenced by dominant biomedical narratives (Woods 122). What Woods brings to the forefront is a need for a further nuancing of these categories that do not allow space for forms that appear incongruent with narrative, such as silence, meaninglessness and formlessness.

In 2013, Seamus O'Mahony published "Against Narrative Medicine," a counterargument to the claims that narrative medicine should be a dominant method of pedagogy for training physicians. O'Mahony argues that "postmodernist literary theory" wrongfully flattens the authority of institutionalized discourse by, for example, understanding a leading article in the *New England Journal of Medicine* and a poem as two equally weighted narratives (612). O'Mahony argues that the intention to teach physicians "empathy" is a task with no measurable outcome. According to the author, it not only risks the physician stepping into a role they are not trained for, such as "spiritual leader," but also cultivates a culture of condemning physicians who cannot or do not desire to grieve with patients. This is an interesting entry point to understand how pushback against narrative medicine starts to grow along seemingly political lines. O'Mahony, for example, makes baffling, uncontextualized claims without citation in his paper such as: "Doctors should—and generally do—treat their patients with courtesy, dignity, and kindness," or "Older, more stoically inclined patients, in particular, may find this form of engagement [empathetic] with their doctor vulgar, embarrassing, and intrusive" (615). He mentions the "grand ambitions" of medical/health humanities as "the promotion of social justice; the teaching of empathy; the encouragement of sensitivity to ethnic, gender, and cultural issues; and an end to the old patriarchalism" (O'Mahony 612). There are overtones in these statements of undermining a perceived softness of social justice perspectives and reinstating the need for the removed, omnipotence of the authoritative institution.

Where some subsequent criticisms of narrative medicine unfold along similar lines, others take a different approach. Mad studies, in particular, has developed a series of criticism of narrative medicine's valorization of Frank's genre typologies and the ways in which mental illness is or is not accounted for. In 2021, Alise de Bie published a review of the literature that examined the outcomes of using autobiographical narratives of madness or mental illness as a pedagogical tool in postsecondary education to teach empathy.

What the author concludes is that the typical approach to using these narratives is a method of colonizing the story of the patient in a way that is highly uncritical of the systems that uphold injustice for Mad communities. Ultimately de Bie finds that intentional engagement with the ethical and epistemological considerations she outlines in the paper can inform how narratives can act as pedagogical tools that may facilitate justice. These considerations include a commitment to foregrounding a critical understanding of how power comes to shape the experiences of Mad people.

Some patient authors have voiced strong criticism of the outcomes of an uncritical narrative medicine. In 2022, Brian Teare wrote an article for *The Boston Review* entitled "Neither Chaos Nor Quest: Toward a Nonnarrative Medicine." Teare calls into question the expectation of patients to earn treatment by relinquishing a redemptive narrative of the self. In critiquing Frank's narrative medicine, Teare notes that while it may appear patient-centred, it ultimately underestimates the influence of the medical-industrial complex and its authorities in allowing patients to express themselves and determining whether their voices are heard. There is no guarantee that these authorities will genuinely listen or comprehend what patients need to be heard. Despite advocating for patient expression and the belief that illness experiences can be articulated, narrative medicine tends to prioritize a specific type of narrative.

Even after recognizing the difficulty patients with chaotic bodies face in narrating their experiences, Teare argues, it still expects them to conform to a particular storytelling model. Teare is speaking about a collision—a collision between what it means for him to be a Queer man with seemingly undiagnosable symptoms in "a taxpayer-funded, city-run public health program for uninsured, low-income residents who made too much income to qualify for Medicare." This collision includes capitalism and his physician, "a butch colluding with patriarchy's classic strategy of gaslighting." A redemptive narrative, for Teare, is out of reach through all the ways in which the factors of his identity, experience, history and pain are incongruent with the healthcare system's "structural inability to interpret non-narrative language as anything but chaos." Ultimately, Teare not only challenges an assumption of the narrative self but also highlights how we have already placed value and meaning on how the story of the patient is understood.

What the collection of works challenging assumptions of narrative medicine can offer this book is two-fold. First, it is significant to separate the various practices and disciplines that are often conflated in the debates outlined in the medical/health humanities, and second, there needs to be a resisting of universal assumptions around the inherent narratology of the self. Medical humanities is a scholarly field that turns to the application of humanities, art and social sciences in medical education and practice. In more recent years a push has been made to rebrand, reimagine, or expand the medical humanities as the health humanities, a strategy to move the academic discipline into a more interdisciplinarity space inclusive of perspectives outside of medicine (Crawford et al. 4). Narrative medicine is a practice that centres the narrative of the patient, typically in medical education or the patient–physician encounter. Narrative therapy, in contrast, is a method for psychological counselling or mental health therapy that uses a distinct framework to develop, deconstruct and reconstruct the life story of the patient as a therapeutic method. Finally, illness narrative is a practice that describes the authorship and presentation of an individual's illness experience. The illness narrative is typically taken-up either textually or verbally (in the case of a patient telling their story to a physician or therapist) but can embody various communicative forms including image and sound. Illness narratives are, at times, misattributed as always existing within, or considered synonymous with, narrative medicine, narrative therapy or medical/health humanities. This is a significant assumption to challenge.

Much of the criticism surrounding medical/health humanities' take-up of narrative medicine either calls into question the ways in which structural power dynamics found in the healthcare system come to exploit the patient's narrative or a sweeping assumption of the self as inherently narrative-bound. While illness narratives are a practice of narrative medicine, they also exist outside the normative healthcare system. This book pushes up against narrative medicine but does not fully intersect. No research is taking place within the walls of the healthcare system, the *Click Me* authors are not framed as patients telling their stories in order to receive better care, and there is no centring of illness narratives as an education tool for physicians alone (the *Click Me* participants do reach a conclusion, though, that their stories should be shared with clinicians and the community for others to learn about their subjective experiences).

This is similar to illness narratives as distinct from narrative therapy. As I argue in "The Possibilities of Illness Narratives in Virtual Reality for Bodies at the Margins":

> Where narrative therapy may require medical professionals to both facilitate the process and measure the outcomes of the therapy, the practice of illness narratives allows for approaches outside, within and parallel to the healthcare system. This is significant for pathologized bodies at the margins, many of whom have experienced subjugation in their healthcare encounters.
>
> (Perram, "The Possibilities of Illness Narratives" 138)

The foundations of the *Click Me* research dislodge the centring of the experience of the reader by removing this position from the study. This research is concerned with the experience of the author and the therapeutic value of the writing process, and displaces the mediation of reading/hearing the narrative (although implications of myself as the researcher reading and analyzing the narratives comes into discussion in Chapter 3). Further, as an extension of reinforcing illness narratives as a practice independent of narrative medicine, this project must resist universal claims regarding the narrative-ness of the self. Illness narratives, specifically in the literary hypertext form, are understood in this book as one response to illness, among many.

## A Note on Narrative Therapy

Illness narratives are deeply tied, in some contexts, to the discipline of narrative therapy. Illness narratives can be one method of narrative therapy, however, writing about one's experience with illness for therapeutic benefit can also be an individualized practice unassociated with any formal stream of therapy. Stephen Madigan argues in the seminal 2019 book, *Narrative Therapy*, that the world view of narrative therapy is one which centres relationality through an anti-individualistic preview. He suggests that this, "relational/contextual/anti-individualist practice was founded on a therapy designed to counter the prevailing dominant psychological ideas regarding the skin-bound individual self" (4). This idea of challenging established belief systems at the core of the skin-bound self, is the foundational core of narrative therapy practice. This practice relies on impartiality and a suspension of judgement from the clinician, where the patient is guided to externalize unhelpful stories from their identity and contextualize values in a way that generates alternative, more productive life stories. Ultimately, this form of therapy encourages the patient to construct stories about their lives as a method to generate meaning from experience.

Narrative therapy was developed by Australian therapist Michael White in his 1990 book *Narrative Means to Therapeutic Ends*, co-authored by David Epston. White's analysis was influenced by the conceptualizations of power dynamics found in feminist, Queer and decolonial theory. White argues that the dominant and established methods and theoretical frameworks for psychology, at the time, involved variations of humanism and structuralism (Madigan 12). Narrative therapy, in contrast, grew in opposition to these methods. White's development of narrative therapy was rooted in the belief that the relational, textual self was influenced by poststructuralist foundational pillars concerned with the relationship between power, identity and knowledge in conjunction with "the origin and location of problems" (Madigan 9). Central to White's conceptualization of narrative therapy was the poststructuralist notion that people are "multi-storied" and experience is nuanced. The therapist, here, acts as a guide to explore and/or challenge the patient's commonly accepted and culturally situated belief systems and how these factors influence thought processes. For narrative therapy, the ways that we come to understand ourselves in relation to the world are limitless and can be "rewritten" in multiple ways.

Parallel to the framework of illness narratives, narrative therapy emerged in response to the dominant discourse at the time that believed the medical/psychological institution housed experts on bodily and mental state, and their knowledge should be gatekept from patients. Narrative therapy, like illness narratives, challenges the process of story relinquishing that can occur in the patient-physician encounter, where the medical institution takes the story of the body and translates it into a highly specialized language, inaccessible to the patient. This story comes to inform a localized, bodily pathology in need of a treatment plan to aid in returning the body to a state of normalcy. For White, the medical institution works to locate and privatize problems as a material site in the body of the patient which upholds beliefs that the body is a docile, subjugated object (Madigan 16). Narrative therapy, in response, uses externalizing conversations to reposition issues "inside the relational and interactional context of culture and discourse, normativity, structural inequalities and so on, and removes the primary site of problems from being privatized inside the decontextualized client body" (Madigan 16).

White was highly influenced by the poststructuralist theories of Michel Foucault in relation to cultural and discursive restraints (Madigan 17), mainly questioning how discourse works to propel "truth" into existence—particularly a patient's "truths" about their identity. In response, narrative therapy would challenge these truths and externalize them as historically informed cultural constructions. Ultimately, meaning about our identities, experiences and relationships is mediated through the process of how, and through what means, we tell our stories. These stories hold real power over and through our relationality with the world. Narrative therapy suggests stories of the self can be told in multiple ways, which in turn, is a generative process for conflicting truths. Narrative therapy scholars Brown and Augusta-Scott argue narrative therapy refutes perspectives of former therapy frameworks that function from the belief that there is an untouched, true essence of the self and that therapy is the practice of emancipating this self. Narrative therapy situates the self, in contrast, as a subject constructed through, and inseparable from, historical, political and social forces. Brown and Augusta-Scott argue that narrative therapy is emerging from this vantage point that "modernist" perspectives of therapy are flawed as they are uncritical of their discursive practice that reinforces dominant ideologies regarding morality: it is universally right to be a certain way and adhering to this will mandate emotional well-being.

Brown and Augusta-Scott write that "discourse of the therapeutic idea pervades daily life" in that it shapes how we interact with the world and forms our identities (8). Through "modernist" therapeutic perspectives, this shaping makes ideological decisions regarding how we function in a social order and what we deem as appropriate behaviour in a cultural context. The authors note that narrative therapy is mirroring former methods of therapy in that it claims it will "help" a patient feel better. However, the disruption of narrative therapy comes from its departure from "modernist" forms of therapies' stance that therapy is ahistorical and apolitical. The authors note:

> We believe that while therapy can indeed invoke conservatizing, normalizing, and regulating processes of self in its operation as a social strategy of power, it can also be an effort to challenge the discursive practices of power and knowledge that have become problematically embedded within people's lives.
>
> (9)

In narrative therapy, it is believed that modifying an individual's life story can bring about change in their actual life. This involves challenging dominant social narratives that emerge in the patient's problem-laden stories about themselves and their lives. It is acknowledged within this therapeutic approach that all personal narratives are also social narratives and are not the sole product of a single author (9). When dominant social relations of power go unchallenged within these self-narratives, the prevailing assumptions about truth and power are reinforced. Narrative therapy aims to disrupt these dominant discourses which serve to maintain the existing social reality.

From this point, the question of this book is considering how women and nonbinary people with hyperandrogenism can use hypertext technology as a method of narrative therapy to write illness narratives that construct positive relationships between their identities and the world. While this question grounds the content of this book, it also deliberately avoids asking if literary hypertext for hyperandrogenism illness narratives works as a therapeutic tool or not, and this is for several reasons. First the results of the *Click Me* project are not intended to be analyzed as outcomes of a formal therapeutic tool. The *Click Me* Twine module, which will be explored in depth in Chapter 4, is informed by narrative therapy practices, however, illness narratives are viewed as counter-practice to traditional therapy enacted, at times, outside the walls of the medical institution or without monitoring by a therapy professional (Couser, *Recovering Bodies* 4). It is important in this project that the core of the practice of illness narratives remains an act of resistance that can be exercised in isolation.

While this book employs the terms *therapy* and *therapeutic* within the context of the practice of narrative therapy, it also resists labelling aspects of the *Click Me* research as any form of formal, active therapy. This is because therapeutic illness narratives hold an affinity with counter-practice to traditional forms of medical treatment (Couser, *Recovering Bodies* 4). The method is taken up in spaces that lack traditional healthcare resources by individuals who, at times, are seeking alternative methods to address emotional well-being, organize political action and take up space as an identity tied to an "abject" body. The *Click Me* authors did not have contact, at any point during the study, with a psychologist or therapist in relation to the project. Due to illness narrative's sociohistorical marking as a method of political action, it would be inaccurate and a disservice to the *Click Me* authors to tie the practice to any formal therapeutic method. This is not to say that formal therapeutic practices are not or would not be beneficial for individuals with hyperandrogenism. This book merely turns to authors to guide the meaning-making practice following the illness narrative process.

Second, this book begins at a point in the literature where the value of illness narratives has been established, alongside the recognition of literary hypertext as a beneficial outlet of expression for marginalized individuals. At this crux, I am approaching this book at a starting point that understands these two forms as valuable, and from there I seek to explore the nuances of this value for a particular set of individuals. In targeting hypertext's value, space opens up to identify the inverse as well. Through this framework, we can grapple with aspects that did not add value, did not contribute to positive relationship building, or were perceived as inaccessible by the *Click Me* authors.

Ultimately, this book is the legacy of women and individuals sitting at their computer screens, writing their illness stories in blog posts, comment sections, health forums and status updates, in order to individually, or with feedback from the anonymous internet, make meaning from their experiences. A dominant perspective in the literature on narrative therapy, in contrast, understands the practice as a method of psychotherapy administered by a trained therapist (Combs and Freedman 1034). It is significant in this book to uphold the notion of accessibility of illness narratives as a practice of self-expression that can be beneficial inside or beyond institutional walls. Therefore, this book will draw on some aspects of political narrative therapy as one theoretical backdrop to the method of illness narratives, however, the intention will be for illness narrative to remain as counter-practice.

## Chapters Overview

The introductory chapter has been an exploration of the theoretical grounding of illness narratives, using Arthur Frank's *The Wounded Storyteller* as a throughline. Illness can behave as a disruptor that destabilizes the linear narrative we construct about our healthy lives. This experience, ultimately, reveals a latent ableism ingrained within the stories we tell of our *self*. In *the land of the sick*, our experience of the world becomes populated with clinic waiting rooms, researching symptoms, and swallowing medications. Within our new *sick* identity is where our sense of self becomes fundamentally altered. Illness, ultimately, hails a relinquishment of narrative agency to the hegemonic authority of the medical institution. This chapter examines the theoretical foundation of illness narratives. While their therapeutic potential is well established, structural constraints often limit access, particularly for marginalized communities. G. Thomas Couser highlights the transformative power of illness narratives while acknowledging their limitations, which frequently exclude those at the margins. In contrast, literary hypertext is emerging as a method for democratizing access to narrative game design, amplifying voices underrepresented in traditional development. A 2020 project called *Click Me*, engaged ten authors with hyperandrogenism to explore hypertext as a tool for narrative therapy. This research forms the foundation of the book.

Through an interdisciplinary approach that intersects gender studies, medical/health humanities and digital humanities, the subsequent chapters of this book tell a story of how hypertext technology can facilitate narratives of health liberation and contribute to broader social change through education. Chapter 2: "Chemical Messengers: Hyperandrogenism"' traces the intersection of nuances of biological sex embodiment, gender norms, pathologization and the medical treatment and clinical diagnosis hyperandrogenism. It begins with the case of Caster Semenya, a South African Olympian whose athletic success was marred by scrutiny and a subsequent unrelenting investigation of her biological sex. Semenya's existence as an Olympic athlete with sex-based illness has become a focal point for public and legislative discourse around transness and "preserving" women's sports, as well as widespread misconceptions about fairness in sport and the biological factors that determine athletic advantage. The chapter shifts to critical perspectives on discourse, norms and "intersex" bodies in the linguistic turn, drawing from Georges Canguilhem's work on the historical construction of normativity and pathologization, Judith Butler and Michel Foucault's expansions on these foundational ideas, and an analysis of compulsory able-bodiedness and heteronormativity. Finally, the chapter concludes with an "uncanny" look at hyperandrogenism and shows how illness cuts open the temporal self thereby facilitating a need to reconstruct our story in ways that keep our identities and sense of temporality intact.

Chapter 3: "Digital Messengers: Hypertext" situates this project's theoretical lens, feminist new materialism, within the context of the materiality of hypertext theory. It begins with an argument of the central role of matter in the project of hypertext illness narratives. There is something tangible that the materiality of the body brings to our narratives and this book questions what that materiality means and how the material realities of women and nonbinary individuals with hyperandrogenism come to form the digital-material. These meaning-making processes take form through the relationality between code, hormones, hair, flesh, identity and, critically, hypertext. The chapter then outlines the concept of hypertext, tracing its linguistic roots and its evolution through time and within the structure of the internet. The chapter turns to the broader topic of electronic literature, and details the genre's potential beyond traditional narrative forms. Finally, Twine, a software for literary hypertext design, is introduced as a tool that democratizes hypertext writing, providing space for marginalized voices in game development and electronic literature spaces. The chapter concludes by looking at how public discourse addresses issues of sexism and exclusion in game design, ultimately noting the need for safer ways to tell our stories.

Chapter 4: "How to DIY a Hypertext Illness Narrative Module" is a guide for you to build your own hypertext module. This chapter provides a brief description of the *Click Me* study's research design, including the authors' journey through the study and the make-up of the participant group. Emphasizing both theoretical and technical aspects, what follows is a detailed outline of the framework I used to design the narrative therapy-informed Twine illness narrative module which enabled authors to build their own stories about the hyperandrogenous experience. The *Click Me* module detailed in this chapter is intended to serve as a pedagogical tool for clinicians and researchers to design their own modules for patients in need. These patients are envisioned as individuals with hyperandrogenism, but there is also potential in the applications of hypertext therapy for other pathologized identities. Individuals with hyperandrogenism or other nuances of biological sex embodiments, too, who are seeking innovative methods to respond to their illness beyond the normative healthcare system may also find value in this guide.

Chapter 5: "The Abnormal Body" begins with a brief overview of the method of coding the data before turning to the concept of the abnormal body and how this notion becomes centred in the stories of *Click Me* authors. Themes emerge in the narratives of authors including a collective recognition of the first menstruation as the initial moment of "discovering" the abnormality of the body and a perceived dualized abnormality both in the body and mind. The chapter then turns to additional themes explored in the *Click Me* narratives, including the experiences of hyperandrogenous bodies in the healthcare system, empowerment, and how relationships between the author and their community, both construct and deconstruct, the sick identity. This chapter also analyzes narrative perspective and contemplates why each narrative uses the first-person point of view to position the narrator. Finally, it provides insights into what is put forward or left out of the authors' framing of their Twine narratives and shows how authors mediate their stories with external texts and audiences. The narratives in the study uphold a belief system that works to suppress certain counter-discourses such as traditional biomedical approaches, acceptance of abnormality and questioning of the concept of abnormality itself.

Chapter 6: "How Code Makes Meaning or Mapping the Illness Narrative" outlines the embodied materiality of code in forming meaning. This meaning is shaped by factors such as the relationality of digital texts, discourse, content and interactions between readers and authors. The chapter outlines how authors utilized CSS and HTML codes in their Twine stories, using elements like colour, alignment, size and text style to design their narratives to fit a desired aesthetic. This chapter unpacks how seemingly menial design choices made by authors are, in fact, situated in a relational affect with larger discursive forces. This relationality produces meaning through contacts deep inside the interface, alongside the programming structure and beyond the confines of the screen. The chapter moves to explore the crux of this book which is how the *Click Me* authors found Twine impactful for visually mapping and charting their experiences using hyperlinks to ultimately enhance therapeutic reflection. Narrative structure choices made by authors are analyzed to supplement this finding, notably common features such as narrative loops and weaving paths, and how these elements produced affect for the reader/player.

Finally, Chapter 7: "The Future of Digital Illness Narratives" brings into focus the critical need for affordable and accessible methods of supporting individuals with hyperandrogenism, particularly within our current sociopolitical landscape, which not only dehumanizes their experiences through restrictive policies but erases their existence through legislation. We start with the impetus of why hyperandrogenism and why now? The discursive take up of hyperandrogenism in our current moment folds into a larger intersectional political storm that is swirling around erasing transgender identities, threats to gender-affirming care, and policing of women's bodies in sport. Recommendations for future research are discussed in relation to emerging technologies. Here, we turn to look to the future of literary hypertext and illness narratives as a whole and ask the following question: what's next? This chapter comes to a head at the future of illness narrative research and access and ultimately argues that the future is, in fact, here. Diverse digital methods such as social media, games, code, film and VR, are already pushing the conceptual boundaries of what it means to be an author and what it means to tell the story of the body.

Ultimately, the chapters of this book, in differing ways, cycle through a single point: the therapeutic value of writing a literary hypertext illness narrative lies in the distinct process of mapping and charting reflective experiences through hyperlinks accompanied by sharing the narrative with the broader community. To truly cultivate meaningful therapeutic benefits, these narratives should allow both the author and the wider social and medical community to reflect on and understand the subjective experience of illness. This book is a project to point to the transformative potential of literary hypertext technology as a therapeutic tool for writing illness narratives, to encourage the adoption of this practice by those who stand to benefit from it: patients, students, women, the *sick*, nonbinary people, clinicians and you.

## Notes

1 Terms such as "excessive" and "masculinizing" are included in quotation marks as this book questions their perceived cohesiveness.

2 I employ the terms *sick* and *sick identity* throughout this text as a strategy to coax both the generative and restrictive affects of pathologization. *Sick*, and its affects, are seeping in sociohistorical connotations of illness and the ways in which hyperandrogenous bodies are discursively constituted within medicalized frameworks. While the term *sick* may not resonate with all individuals with hyperandrogenism, it serves as a productive framework for this author to speak about bodies that are drawn into discourses of pathology. A more in-depth discussion of the terms *pathology* and *illness* follows in the section "A Note on Language" later in this chapter.

3 I use the term "normative" healthcare system to refer to the standard systems and practices that are institutionalized (privately or publicly) to respond to the health of individuals and communities. In a Canadian context, the normative healthcare system includes institutions such as hospitals and health ministries, healthcare providers, patients and policies that govern the relations between these entities.

4 In this book, the phrase "nuances of biological sex embodiment" will be used to refer to the experience of sex as a spectrum in regard to non-binary manifestations of chromosome patterns, hormones, external genitalia and internal organs. The term "sex-based illness" will be used for pathologization of the "nuances of biological sex embodiment." This pathologizing typically occurs through the classification of differences of sex development (DSD) and as endocrine disorders and conditions, such as hyperandrogenism, that impact hormone production and regulation, as well as the way these two categories intersect. DSD, formerly referred to as "intersex" disorders, are a group of congenital conditions that manifest in utero, in which chromosomal, gonadal or anatomical sex development of the fetus becomes atypical (Cools et al. 415). While hyperandrogenism may intersect with some DSD conditions, it is not inherently labelled as a DSD because it primarily involves hormonal dysregulation rather than structural or chromosomal differences in sex development.

5 I refer to health liberation as a concept of the liberation health framework (see Martinez and Fleck-Henderson) that comes out of social work theory. Liberation health is a method of practice that understands that the seemingly individualized experiences of mental health and illness are, in fact, created in the intersection between social, institutional, economic and political power relations.

6 I refer to the process of embodying gender as a "mode of becoming" in a Butlerian sense where they question: "what happens to gender as a mode of becoming?" (*Undoing Gender* 81) when our norms for care work to cement bodies into fixed binaries.

7 See section below entitled "A Note on Language" regarding the language choice of "self-identify" rather than "diagnosed."

8 The decision to centre the disease PCOS over hyperandrogenism in the recruitment of this study is explained in depth in Chapter 4.

9 A description of the Twine software, its origins, and its enduring influence as counter-practice is detailed in Chapter 3, within the section titled "Twinery.org."

10 As discussed in an earlier footnote of this chapter, the term "intersex" has been largely replaced in medical contexts with the term DSD. However, this book intentionally retains the use of "intersex" in specific moments when contextualizing the social space around hyperandrogenism discourse.

**Works Cited**


Anthony, Kate, and DeeAnna Merz Nagel. *Therapy Online: A Practical Guide*. SAGE, 2010.

Anthropy, Anna. *Rise of the Videogame Zinesters: How Freaks, Normals, Amateurs, Artists, Dreamers, Dropouts, Queers, Housewives, and People Like You Are Taking Back an Art Form*, 1st ed. Seven Stories Press, 2012.

Bazarganipour, Fatemeh, et al. “Health-Related Quality of Life and Its Relationship with Clinical Symptoms Among Iranian Patients with Polycystic Ovarian Syndrome.” *Iranian Journal of Reproductive Medicine*, vol. 11, no. 5, 2013, pp. 371–378.

Battersby, James L. “Narrativity, Self, and Self-Representation.” *Narrative*, vol. 14, no. 1, 2006, pp. 27–44.

Bolaki, Stella. *Illness as Many Narratives: Arts, Medicine and Culture*. Edinburgh University Press, 2016.

Brown, Catrina and Tod Augusta-Scott, editors. *Narrative Therapy: Making Meaning, Making Lives*. SAGE Publications, Inc., 2007.

Butler, Judith. *Bodies That Matter: On the Discursive Limits of “Sex”*. Routledge, 2011.

Butler, Judith. *Undoing Gender*. Routledge, 2004, pp. 40–56.

Combs, Gene, and Jill Freedman. “Narrative, Poststructuralism, and Social Justice: Current Practices in Narrative Therapy.” *The Counseling Psychologist*, vol. 40, no. 7, 2012, pp. 1033–1060.

Cools, Martine, et al. “Caring for Individuals with a Difference of Sex Development (DSD): A Consensus Statement.” *Nature Reviews Endocrinology*, vol. 14, 2018, pp. 415–429.

Couser, G. Thomas. “Disability, Life Narrative, and Representation.” *PMLA*, vol. 120, no. 2, 2005, pp. 602–606.

Couser, G. Thomas. *Recovering Bodies: Illness, Disability, and Life Writing*. University of Wisconsin Press, 1997.

Couser, G. Thomas. *Signifying Bodies: Disability in Contemporary Life Writing*. University of Michigan Press, 2009.

Couser, G. Thomas. *Vulnerable Subjects: Ethics and Life Writing*. Cornell University Press, 2004.

Cousin, Norman. *Anatomy of an Illness as Perceived by the Patient: Reflections on Healing and Regeneration*. Bantam Books, 1979.

Crawford, Paul, et al. “Health Humanities: The Future of Medical Humanities?” *Mental Health Review Journal*, vol. 15, no. 3, 2010, pp. 4–10.

Davis, Georgiann, and Sharon Preves. “Intersex and the Social Construction of Sex.” *Contexts*, vol. 16, no. 1, 2017, p. 80.

de Bie, Alise. “Teaching with Madness/‘Mental Illness’ Autobiographies in Postsecondary Education: Ethical and Epistemological Implications.” *Medical Humanities*, vol. 48, no. 1, 2021, pp. 37–50.

Dumaresque, Renee, et al. “Politicized Narrative Therapy: A Reckoning and a Call to Action.” *Canadian Social Work Review/Revue Canadienne de Service Social*, vol. 35, no. 1, 2018, pp. 109–129.

Ensslin, Astrid. *Writing New Bodies*. Project website, 2019, https://sites.google.com/ualberta.ca/writingnewbodies/home.

Fausto-Sterling, Anne. “The Five Sexes: Why Male and Female Are Not Enough.” *Sciences*, vol. 33, 1993, pp. 20–20.

Frank, Arthur W. *The Wounded Storyteller: Body, Illness, and Ethics*, 2nd ed. The University of Chicago Press, 2013.

Graham, Connor, et al. "Blogging as 'Therapy'? Exploring Personal Technologies for Smoking Cessation." *Health Informatics Journal*, vol. 15, no. 4, 2009, pp. 267–281.

Hawkins, Anne Hunsaker. *Reconstructing Illness: Studies in Pathography*. Purdue University Press, 1993.

htr12. "Breaking Down Emotionally Over PCOS." *SoulCysters*, 21 March 2015, http://soulcysters.com/here-we-go-my-story/#. Accessed 1 August 2017.

Irvine, Craig, and Rita Charon. "Deliver Us from Certainty: Training for Narrative Ethics." *The Principles and Practice of Narrative Medicine*, edited by Rita Charon et al., Oxford University Press, 2017, pp. 110–136.

Karjula, Salla, et al. "Psychological Distress Is More Prevalent in Fertile Age and Premenopausal Women with PCOS Symptoms: 15-Year Follow-Up." *Journal of Clinical Endocrinology & Metabolism*, vol. 102, no. 6, 2017, pp. 1861–1869, doi:10.1210/jc.2016-3863.

Kelly, Christine, and Michael Orsini. "Beyond Measure? Disability Art, Affect and Reimagining Visitor Experience." *Studies in Social Justice*, vol 15, no. 2, 2021, pp. 288–306.

Kleinman, Arthur. *The Illness Narratives: Suffering, Healing, and the Human Condition*. Basic Books, 1988.

Klimas, Chris. *Twine*. The Interactive Technology Foundation, 2009, http://twinery.org/.

Lear, Martha Weinman. *Heartsounds*. Simon & Schuster, 1980.

Lucidi, Richard Scott, Ed. "Polycystic Ovarian Syndrome Clinical Presentation." *Medscape*, 2016.

Mackenzie, Catriona and Jacqui Poltera. "Narrative Integration, Fragmented Selves, and Autonomy." *Hypatia*, vol. 25, no. 1, 2020, pp. 32–54.

Madigan, Stephen. *Narrative Therapy*, 2nd ed. American Psychological Association, 2019.

Martinez, Dawn Belkin, and Ann Fleck-Henderson. *Social Justice in Clinical Practice: A Liberation Health Framework for Social Work*. Routledge, 2014.

O'Mahony, Seamus. "Against Narrative Medicine." *Perspectives in Biology and Medicine*, vol. 56, no. 4, 2013, pp. 611–619.

Perram, Megan, and Astrid Ensslin. "The Possibilities of Illness Narratives in Virtual Reality for Bodies at the Margins." *Digital Creativity*, vol. 33, no. 2, 2022, pp. 128–156.

Perram, Megan, and Astrid Ensslin. *Soul Cysters Dot Net: Configuring the Feminine Body Through the Life Writing of Women with Polycystic Ovarian Syndrome*. 2017. University of Alberta, Master's Capstone. *Education & Research Archive*.

Phelan, James. "Editor's Column: Who's Here? Thoughts on Narrative Identity and Narrative Imperialism." *Narrative*, vol. 13, no. 3, 2005, pp. 205–210.

Rains, Steve. *Coping with Illness Digitally*. MIT Press, 2018.

Schechtman, Marya. "Stories, Lives, and Basic Survival: A Refinement and Defense of the Narrative View." *Narrative and Understanding Persons*, edited by Daniel D. Hutto, Cambridge University Press, 2007, pp. 155–178.

Schippers, Mimi. "Recovering the Feminine Other: Masculinity, Femininity, and Gender Hegemony." *Theory and Society*, vol. 36, no. 1, 2007, pp. 85–102.

Stryker, Susan, and Stephen Whittle, eds. *The Transgender Studies Reader*. Routledge, 2013.

Sterling, E. W., et al. "A Study of Perceptions, Experiences, and Satisfaction with Healthcare among Women with Polycystic Ovary Syndrome (PCOS)." *Fertility and Sterility*, vol. 94, no. 4, Supplement S7, September 2010.

Strawson, Galen. "Against Narrativity." *Ratio*, vol. 17, no. 4, 2004, pp. 428–452.

Sulik, Gayle A. "'Our Diagnoses, Our Selves': The Rise of the Technoscientific Illness Identity." *Sociology Compass*, vol. 5, no. 6, 2011, pp. 463–477.

Svenaeus, Fredrik. "The Body Uncanny—Further Steps Towards a Phenomenology of Illness." *Medicine, Health Care and Philosophy*, vol. 3, 2000, pp. 125–137.

Tammi, Pekka. "Against Narrative ('A Boring Story')." *Partial Answers: Journal of Literature and the History of Ideas*, vol. 4, no. 2, 2006, pp. 19–40.

Teare, Brian. "Neither Chaos Nor Quest: Toward a Nonnarrative Medicine." *The Boston Review*, 3 February 2022, https://www.bostonreview.net/articles/neither-chaos-nor-quest-toward-a-nonnarrative-medicine/#:~:text=Narrative%20medicine%20claims%20to%20champion,what%20is%20wrong%20with%20them. Accessed 5 December 2022.

White, Michael, and David Epston. *Narrative Means to Therapeutic Ends*. Norton, 1990.

Woods, Angela. "Beyond the Wounded Storyteller: Rethinking Narrativity, Illness and Embodied Self-Experience." *Health, Illness and Disease*, edited by Havi Carel and Rachel Cooper, Routledge, 2013, pp. 125–140.

Yildiz, Bulent O. "Diagnosis of Hyperandrogenism: Clinical Criteria." *Best Practice & Research: Clinical Endocrinology & Metabolism*, vol. 20, no. 2, 2006, pp. 167–176.

# 2 Chemical Messengers
## Hyperandrogenism

### Cultural Take-Up of Hyperandrogenism

Hyperandrogenism and other nuances of biological sex embodiment have been employed as a justification to call into question which bodily signifiers and hormonal nuances quantify biological sex. A relatively understudied and socially stigmatized condition, hyperandrogenism has recently gained media attention as the focal point of the "sex verification testing" Olympic controversy. Following the public dispute over South African track runner Caster Semenya's 2009 gold medal in the 800 meters at the World Championships, she was mandated by the International Association of Athletics Federations (IAAF) to undergo a "sex-verification" test. The general secretary of the IAAF requested the verification of eligibility on the same day she had won the gold medal due to "ambiguity" regarding her biological sex (Cooky and Dwarkin 103). The results of the sex test were never officially published, however, certain findings were leaked to the media and subsequently widely debated, leading to unverified claims regarding Semenya potentially possessing an "intersex" diagnosis.

Media coverage at the time speculated the sex inquiry was made specifically because of the deeper register of Semenya's voice, her muscular build and her stark race time improvement (Cooky and Dwarkin 103). Subsequent reports noted that Semenya has been diagnosed with the condition 5-alpha-reductase 2 deficiency, resulting in natural testosterone levels within the typical male range (Ingle). Semenya was raised as a girl and has always identified as a woman. Amidst the divide of a deeply contested cultural landscape, Semenya stood at the forefront in 2023, writing an opinion piece titled "Running in a Body That's My Own" for *The New York Times*. Defiantly, Semenya writes,

> I know I look like a man. I know I sound like a man and maybe even walk like a man and dress like one, too. But I'm not a man; I'm a woman. Playing sports and having muscles and a deep voice make me less feminine, yes. I'm a different kind of woman, I know, but I'm still a woman.
> ("Running in a Body")

DOI: 10.4324/9781003646921-2

The IAAF came up against significant criticism regarding its treatment of Caster Semenya following the 2009 World Championships, which prompted a call to review and assess the organization's "sex verification" protocols. In May 2011, as a response to these calls to action, the IAAF implemented the "Regulations Governing Eligibility of Females with Hyperandrogenism to Compete in Women's Competition." These regulations were put into place to manage cases where the sex of an athlete was being publicly contested, paying particular attention to women embodying real or suspected hyperandrogenism. At the time, individuals diagnosed with hyperandrogenism were mandated to inform the IAAF, while at the same time, the IAAF's medical manager was given authority to "investigate" suspected cases of hyperandrogenism, which was contingent on what was called "reasonable grounds" (Wu). The testosterone levels of these athletes had to remain below the 10 nmol/L threshold in order to participate, or, the athlete had to demonstrate androgen resistance, which was justified as a quantifiable threshold to negate any potential competitive advantage. Ultimately, adhering to these regulations often required athletes to seek prescriptions for anti-androgen medications or pursue surgical interventions (Wu).

The Court of Arbitration for Sport (CAS), which is an international body that works to settle sports disputes through arbitration, came to a decision, in 2015, to suspend the implementation of the 2011 regulations for a period of two years due to a legal challenge brought forward by an Indian sprinter named Dutee Chand. CAS's verdict was based on the conclusion that the IAAF had failed to substantiate the nature of the regulations in ensuring equity within women's athletics. Ultimately, CAS found that the IAAF were not able to provide empirical evidence demonstrating that hyperandrogenism produces a distinct significant athletic advantage (Wu). From this verdict, the IAAF was given a two-year window to bring forward evidence to support their conclusion, which they did not. Instead, the IAAF opted to replace the 2011 regulations with a new set of 2018 Eligibility Regulations. The new regulations targeted female athletes who embodied DSD and/or testosterone levels exceeding a threshold of 5 nmol/L, a new standard that was notably lower than what was set in previous regulations (Wu). Semenya formally challenged the new regulations in June 2018 where her legal team argued that the new regulations violate multiple legal frameworks, including the IAAF Constitution, the Olympic Charter, Monaco's laws, and globally recognized human rights (Wu). CAS dismissed Semeny's challenge in May of 2019 which permitted the new regulations to take effect. CAS, at this time, acknowledged that while the regulations were, in fact, discriminatory, this discrimination was "a necessary, reasonable, and proportionate means of achieving the IAAF's aim of preserving the integrity of female athletics" (Ingle).

Semenya then took her appeal to the Federal Supreme Court of Switzerland. The court provisionally suspended the World Athletics rules while considering whether to issue an interlocutory injunction, however, this decision was reversed, leaving Semenya unable to compete in World Athletics races between 400 meters and one mile while her appeal continued. The Swiss Supreme Court ultimately rejected Semenya's appeal in September 2020. The court, in its decision, noted that CAS had the right to uphold World Athletics' regulation "in order to guarantee fair competition for certain running disciplines in female athletics" (Mather).

The next year Semenya appealed her case to the European Court of Human Rights. Parallel to this appeal, in March 2023, World Athletics began to implement more robust regulations for individuals with DSD. The new rules mandate that these athletes must lower their testosterone levels below a threshold of 2.5 nmol/L for a minimum of 24 months before being eligible to compete (Spary). In July 2023, the European Court of Human Rights heard Semenya's appeal and ultimately ruled in her favour with a 4–3 decision. The court found that the implementation of these new rules had, in fact, discriminated against Semenya and others like her, and infringed on her human rights. While validating Semenya's experiences, this ruling did not have the authority to overturn the regulations themselves, and World Athletics upheld their regulations. The Swiss government requested that Semenya's case be referred to the European Court of Human Rights' Grand Chamber in November 2023 for a final ruling ("Semenya Case Referred to European Rights Court's Grand Chamber"). On May 15, 2024, the Grand Chamber hearing for the case of Semenya v. Switzerland began and, at the time of writing this book, the implications are still pending.

Encapsulated within the Olympic "sex-verification test" controversy are overtones of racism. As Zine Magubane argues in their article "Spectacles and Scholarship: Caster Semenya, Intersex Studies, and the Problem of Race in Feminist Theory," the process of Semenya's formation as an "intersex" subject through institutional regulation holds within it, a racially contingent qualifier. The author argues that

> even when the idea that the truth of sex is anchored in the body is thrown radically into doubt, race still provides an anchor…From the seventeenth century onward, race overdetermined whether bodies in doubt needed to be resolved and how that resolution would take place.
>
> (781)

The ways in which the caricature of Semenya is constructed in public discourse is predicated on her race where she becomes not a body obscured in her biological sex presentation, but an unreadable Black body from the Global South. The caricature created from Semenya's likeness, in this sense, becomes the representing narrative through which sport economies of the Global North and South play out allowing for relentless regulation, surveillance, testing, trials, documentation and modification of the racialized body.

In court documents, the IAAF is quoted as saying: "There are some contexts where biology has to trump identity" (The Associated Press). The stance of IAAF, however, is predicated on several significant misconceptions. According to authors Cheryl Cooky and Shari L. Dworkin in their article "Policing the Boundaries of Sex: A Critical Examination of Gender Verification and the Caster Semenya Controversy," three grave misconceptions that underpin IAAF's perspective are the following: biological sex is a dualistic binary, sports competitions are already level playing fields for those who compete, and elevated testosterone gives women a distinct athletic advantage (103). The IAAF's regulations fail to account for the complex interplay of biological factors that contribute to athletic performance, as well as deeply impactful social factors, and instead attribute disproportionate importance to testosterone levels. This is a relative dominant assumption that overlooks the multifaceted nature of athleticism, which includes a variety of physiological, psychological and environmental factors. Ultimately, IAAF's policies are based on an oversimplified and scientifically contested understanding of the relationship between testosterone and competitive advantage.

Beyond the results of the "sex-verification" test, Semenya has detailed her experiences over the years of being mandated to undergo intrusive, humiliating and dehumanizing examinations from the age of 18 (The Associated Press). Semenya's experience of hyperandrogenism, and many other women competing in professional and amateur sports, has included a public defence of their biological sex as well as their gender identity and sexuality. Semenya's story invokes the experiences of women, transgender individuals and those with DSD whose identities in sport have been contested on the public stage, including, for example, the stories of María José Martínez-Patiño, Imar Khalid, Lin Yu-Ting, Dutee Chand and Christine Mboma.

## The Pathologization of Hyperandrogenism

As discussed in earlier chapters of this book, hyperandrogenism is a prevalent expression of PCOS, the most common endocrine disorder for women of childbearing age (Badawy and Elnashar 25). Hyperandrogenism is a complex diagnosis because it appears as a display of symptoms that could be tied to several underlying sex-based illnesses including PCOS, Congenital Adrenal Hyperplasia, or Cushing's syndrome, among others (Rachoń 205). Medical literature affirms that disordered causes of hyperandrogenism may be medically critical but choosing not to treat elevated testosterone for some women may pose "no health risk" (Sonksen et al. 826). In clinical practice, women diagnosed with hyperandrogenism are prescribed anti-androgens or else advised of cosmetic “solutions” including laser hair removal, medication for male-pattern hair loss, and bleaching cream to “restore” feminine embodiment (Cannon 15).

*Medscape*, a dominant online medical resource for educating physicians and healthcare practitioners on clinical guidelines, offers peer-reviewed scholarly guides on the presentation and treatment of diseases, including hormonal disorders. The description of hyperandrogenism’s presentation on *Medscape* produces a clear pathologizing of bodies that deviate from normative gender embodiment. PCOS clinical guidelines call for physicians to conduct a visual exam for increased testosterone. The modified Ferriman–Gallwey (mFG) score grades nine areas of the body from 0 (no hair) to 4, “including the upper lip, chin, chest, upper abdomen, lower abdomen, thighs, back, arm, and buttocks” (Lucidi). *Medscape* notes that “a total score of 8 or more is considered abnormal for an adult white woman”. The modified Ferriman–Gallwey (mFG) score, particularly in the way it is described here, is insufficient for various reasons. These guidelines fail to provide further context regarding the different criteria for white women versus non-white women and how this difference should be interpreted, direction on informed consent for the patient in regards to the visual examination, methods for uniform interpretation of the degree of “excess” hair, and how to screen for permanent or non-permanent hair removal practices that may have already been done on the body prior to the exam.

When visual cues for elevated testosterone are a diagnostic tool, the cause for medical concern would arise in the appearance of hirsutism where “hair is commonly seen on the upper lip, on the chin, around the nipples, and along the linea alba of the lower abdomen” (Lucidi). For physicians, visual symptoms of “abnormality” in diagnosing increased testosterone would also include signs of male-pattern baldness, clitoromegaly (enlarged clitoris), increased muscle mass, acne and deepening voice (Lucidi). Some women diagnosed with PCOS are given options of “medical treatment” for “excess” facial and body hair growth, suggesting, in conjunction with weight loss, “shaving and the use of chemical depilatories and/or bleaching cream” may be used (Lucidi). The clinical guidelines go on to explain that because plucking or waxing may cause ingrown hairs, “long-term, more permanent measures for unwanted hairs include electrolysis and laser treatment” (Lucidi). Within the framework of this diagnostic language, it is the display of gender deviation that is pathologized (such as “masculine” features, infertility, and abnormal menstruation), rather than the underlying source of dysfunction (if one is present). The insufficiency of both PCOS diagnostic criteria and clinical procedures is two-fold. First, the centring of “androgen excess” which focuses on clinical signs of “increased” male hormones as a diagnostic criterion indicates a pathologizing of the bodies of women with PCOS that deviate from normative gender embodiment.

As I argue in "Illness of the Gendered Body, Freud's *The Uncanny*, and 'Being-in-the-World,'" the institutional treatment of hyperandrogenism is an act of medical and cultural pathologizing of deviant femininity. The pathology, in this sense, contributes to perceptions of abnormality in women with hyperandrogenism. Women with hyperandrogenism "because they fail by cultural standards to embody normative femininity—perceive themselves as reduced to a dysfunctional body, an abnormal body, and a body that must be treated medically" (Perram 3). This is a finding that is echoed in the literature on the experiences of women with PCOS (Ekback et al. 358; Himelein and Thatcher 613; Yoo et al. 3; Pfister and Rømer 167). According to some experiences, as told through illness narratives depicting the clinical encounter, hyperandrogenism becomes coded as a failing of hegemonic femininity. Here, an idea is born that once one is able to "achieve" a normative body, one will, in fact, be "cured" of the disease (Perram 3). This narrative not only ignores the potential concern of "root causes" of hyperandrogenism but also reinforces misconceptions of a biological sex binary (see Fausto-Sterling).

The question, here, is where do women go if they are not finding value in the medical encounter? Recent literature suggests that women with PCOS are dissatisfied with the diagnostic process and therefore are seeking information through alternative sources (Hoyos et al.). In a study conducted by Gibson-Helm et al. it was found that in a sample size of 1385 women, only 35.2% were satisfied with their diagnosis experience. The main reasons for dissatisfaction, according to authors, were delayed diagnosis and inadequate information (Gibson-Helm et al. 604). The most critical area that women in the study believed required improvement was effective educational materials. Participants in the study identified forums, workshops, emails and informational websites as potentially effective methods of education dissemination to patients during the diagnosis experience (608). Further, this study illuminates a distinct issue around access to a diagnosis. The authors note that, on average, women in their study encountered over three health professionals over the duration of one year in order to receive a diagnosis of PCOS (Gibson-Helm et al. 608). It must be noted that a lengthy process with multiple contacts with clinicians would not inherently be a negative experience for all patients, however, it is telling that participants identified this process as inadequate. It is the substance of these encounters that appears to be lacking where patients yearn for meaningful connections with the healthcare system that ultimately better equips them to live with their illness.

This particular study did not focus on diverging experiences of diagnosis for Women of Colour. Women of Colour experience PCOS more intensely and frequently than white women (Basile). PCOS commonly has comorbidities or a high frequency of presenting itself with one or more other diseases and/or medical conditions. Most of these comorbidities, such as metabolic syndrome, also affect Women of Colour more drastically. Black and Latinx communities have higher morbidity and mortality rates due to cardiovascular disease and diabetes and Black women and Mexican communities have higher rates of hyperinsulinemia and insulin resistance (Basile). The emergence of health disparities that arise along racial lines is formed by social and environmental racism and oppression. For example, Black women with PCOS experience higher rates of hirsutism, obesity and infertility compared to white women, yet have poorer access to fertility treatments (Galic et al. 109). PCOS and hyperandrogenism, like many diseases, are race and class issues. The narratives of the *Click Me* authors, which are examined in detail in subsequent chapters, provide profound insights into how racial and class disparities influence the diagnosis, treatment and management of PCOS and hyperandrogenism.

## Discourse, Norms and "Intersex" Bodies in the Linguistic Turn

Coming into contact with the cultural discourse surrounding hyperandrogenous embodiment is a theoretical evolution grappling with a deceptively complex question: What does it mean to be *sick*? When grappling with "intersex" identity through feminist theory, conceptualizations of norms, normalization, and pathologization are foundational. Georges Canguilhem's *The Normal and the Pathological* has endured as a seminal text tracing the historical lineage of biological notions of *normal* and deviance into *pathological*. Canguilhem plots the early 19th-century conceptualizations of health and disease and demonstrates how the emergent epistemological bases of normal and pathological were politically, economically and institutionally supported. Rather than biological, essentialist categories, Canguilhem shapes a radical philosophy that rejects a statistical certainty of the normal in favour of qualitative valuation. Canguilhem shows how pathology through bodily dysfunction is tied to a failure to adapt to the ever-evolving state of the normal and therefore cannot be separated from the experience or judgement of the individual. Canguilhem's work has gone on to influence the philosophies of many prominent theorists, shaping the ways in which they view the evolution of knowledge through history and the turbulent practice of establishing pillars of truth. Drawing from the work of Canguilhem, Judith Butler and Michel Foucault have formed the basis of their philosophies on a notion of *normal* as that which conforms to a norm and the *pathological* as a value description of the space outside the fluctuating boundary of the normal.

Critical to establishing the theoretical foundation of this book is an engagement with poststructuralist theory and sexuality studies, particularly in examining how these perspectives conceptualize "intersex" bodies as being regulated through discourse. Decades of feminist theory on discursive (re)production of the body have been preceded by the work of Michel Foucault. In 1975, Foucault published the landmark *Discipline and Punish: The Birth of the Prison*. In this work, Foucault discusses his concept of docile bodies where he argues that the subject is produced through normalized forms of surveillance and disciplinary power. The docility of the body is achieved through its regulation in a particular time and space. Foucault discusses the assemblages of subjects in space through the context of the institution. The societal institution takes many forms but includes the school, the prison, the military and the hospital. Through combinations of series, subjects are placed in confined sequences (military ranks, students in a classroom or prisoners in cells) and subjected to constant, elusive surveillance (i.e., the Panopticon). Docile bodies are also produced through the regulation of personal, economic, political and historical time in order to govern the way in which the subject experiences the passing of intervals. According to Foucault, the combined, coercive ownership of the subject's body in both time and space works to manipulate the subject as docile. Because the power of this organizational practice is productive and codified, these coercive measures are normalized and therefore indiscernible.

In 1976, Foucault laid the groundwork for contemporary feminist sexuality studies through the publication of *The History of Sexuality*. Foucault takes a sociohistorical approach to the production of sexuality as a concept arguing that it is through sex's discursive rendering as a site of power that the concept is born in the first place. As sexuality continued to infiltrate institutional discursive dynamics (through its perception as a cultural taboo, for example), it began to erect itself as an entity of subjecthood. Foucault concludes that when we are able to dissolve the discursive form of sexuality in our cultural, institutional and political assemblages we will truly become liberated from the oppression our ideas of sexuality place on identity. Foucault challenges the "repressive hypothesis" that argues power regulations have historically worked to repress the discussion of sexuality. Foucault suggests it is through historical regulation of sex, from the practice of Christian confession to tightening laws on "deviant" sex acts, that sexuality became a frequent topic in public discourse. Once sex became discursive, conceptions of a normal and pathological sexuality were produced. In this sense, Foucault argues that power is not, in fact, repressive, but productive.

Power produces subject positions, and in the case of the historical swelling of discursive sexuality, sexuality became an identity category and central to the ways in which we understood and spoke about ourselves and our communities. This productive form of power that has birthed discursive sexuality, according to Foucault, also generates a way to speak and know about deviant sexuality. We see this in the varying ways that sexuality in relation to children, same-sex partners, multiple partners, labour and commodification, consent and animals has been criminalized or pathologized throughout time. Foucault's work on discourse at the site of power and his poststructuralist theoretical approach have gone on to form the foundation of prominent streams of gender and Queer studies to date as well as conceptualizations of illness subjectivities. Foucault's legacy intersects with the experience of hyperandrogenism through the ways in which we understand how medicalized discourse comes to shape illness and the process of pathologizing the abnormal, abject body.

In 1980, Julia Kristeva wrote *Powers of Horror: An Essay on Abjection*, a poststructuralist and psychoanalytic exploration of the concept of the abject, building on the traditional theories of Sigmund Freud and Jacques Lacan. Kristeva argues that the abject is the feeling of subjective horror and disgust that is experienced by the confrontation of the *self* with the *other*. This recognition of distinct subject positions makes us aware of our own corporeal reality and creates a feeling of incongruence. The abject, then, is a subjective realization of the *other*, or that which is not a part of the *self*. Further, the abject is situated outside of the ways in which we organize categories, and therefore a confrontation with the abject jars our methods of conceptualization. For instance, Kristeva turns to examples of garbage, filth or a human corpse. These entities were once subjects in our cultural order but have now been "cast off" outside our realm of subjecthood. Yet, we can still recognize them in our environment, and this is what produces cognitive dissonance. This sense of incongruence triggers a desire to reproduce organizational boundaries to maintain our relationship with logical subjecthood. This desire is typically enacted through rituals that work to create a sense of separation from nature and society. Kristeva's analysis of the abject has gone on to influence a host of disciplines, including disability and gender studies.

In *Disability Studies: An Interdisciplinary Introduction*, Dan Goodley argues that the social and human sciences have historically constructed the concept of the "individual with impairments" through disciplinary power relations that reinforce neoliberal ideals of productivity, independence, and self-sufficiency (p. 66). Goodley calls into question the process of "psychologizing" disability and asks us to contend with how psychology has played a central role in shaping normative understandings of personhood by legitimizing statistical norms, reinforcing eugenicist classifications and upholding the ideological values of capitalist modernity. Goodley suggests that the emergence of the "average individual" as a standard against which all bodies are measured has led to the marginalization of those deemed "abnormal," positioning disability as a deviation from the socially constructed ideal of the able-bodied citizen (p. 69). By pulling apart the tensions that which entangle psychology, capitalism and biopolitics, ultimately what we are left with is a challenging of

Western hegemonic frameworks that situate disability, and by extension, illness, as an individualized "problem" (p. 70).

Gender scholars such as Judith Butler have turned to the concept of the abject body to understand how bodies that challenge our normative binaries create a sense of cultural panic. Judith Butler discusses the concept of the abject body in her book 1996 *Bodies That Matter*. According to Butler, the abject body refers to bodies that deviate from a cultural understanding of the sex binary and therefore become excluded from the normative standards of society. Butler uses the concept of the abject to describe how, through regulatory systems, bodies are filtered into a binary of normal and deviant. The abject body, then, becomes simultaneously a site of anxiety and fascination for the dominant culture because it takes hold of, and makes coherent, a space outside of normativity. The dominant culture processes the abject body as something both threatening and attractive as it exposes the limits of the constructed nature of gender. The concept of the abject body is critical to understand the experience hyperandrogenism and is a term that this book relies on to explore the drive, from the self, from culture and institutionally, to "cure" the hyperandrogenous body by pushing it back into the normative category of the feminine.

For "intersex" bodies, Canguilhem's legacy of norms and pathologization becomes significant when evaluating the concept of sex dimorphism and a sex binary in humans. A pivotal text in feminist science studies is Anne Fausto-Sterling's 1993 article "The Five Sexes: Why Male and Female Are Not Enough" where she argues that categories of male and female are not sufficient to capture the nuances of human sexual biology. Fausto-Sterling argues that in "nature" there is evidence for five distinct sexes. Feminist sex theory today has built on Fausto-Sterling's claims shining a light on the myriad of "naturally" produced "intersex" identities that may render variances in sex chromosomes, hormones, external genital and internal organs. For the *Click Me* authors—women and nonbinary individuals with hyperandrogenism who are at times labelled as "intersex" (as seen in news coverage on Caster Semenya)—Canguilhem's theory illuminates a connection between how hyperandrogenous bodies become pathologized through medicalized discourse.

In 1993, Deborah Findlay wrote the ground-breaking article "Discovering Sex: Medical Science, Feminism and Intersexuality" that reinforced Anne Fausto-Sterling's argument of biological sex multiplicity in "The Five Sexes." Findlay maps the definitional categories of biological sex both employed and produced by obstetrician–gynaecologists in the 1950s Canada. Findlay looks at how scientific practices of medicine are actually proponents of sociology in the way that they work to produce social concepts of biological sex. The field of medical science, according to Findlay, then weaponizes these social concepts as naturalized "proof" of dichotomized sex. This in turn leads to a presumed distinction between social understandings of sex and gender and scientific understandings that allows for the pathologization of deviant sex (Findlay 26). Instances of "natural" "intersex" bodies are then able to be framed as "abnormal" and a quest to "discover" the "true" sex of the body becomes the mission of medical care.

Findlay's study looks at the decade of the 1950s as this was when the genetic test for the nuclear sex chromatin was discovered and became used as an instrument to "decipher" the "true" biological sex of ambiguously sexed infants. The discovery of the genetic test superseded previous methods of sex verification in medicine, including gonadal and hormonal tests (Findlay 36). This genetic test for the nuclear sex chromatin was a significant and timely discovery because it came at a time where an infant's ambiguous external genitalia was viewed as a medical emergency. This is a sentiment that is very much true today as clinicians felt and continue to feel institutionalized pressure to pronounce biological sex at birth via the birth certificate. Findlay analyzed a sample of ten prominent obstetrician–gynaecologist textbooks to examine not only the medicalized discourse on the pages, but the "metaphors, illustrations, and taken-for-granted assumptions about female biology" that contributed to the fallacy of a sex binary (34). Findlay concludes "Sex, then, was not 'biological material' waiting to be discovered in nature; rather, it was a representation, embodying specific assumptions about what biological sex should be like" (44). This is an important ontological starting point for our understanding of hyperandrogenism to approach biological sex as produced through and enforced by ourselves in relationship with medicalized discourse. In this way, the pathologizing of deviant biological sex found in the experience of hyperandrogenism can easily be linked to other sex-based illnesses such as "intersex" disorder, Congenital Adrenal Hyperplasia, testosterone biosynthetic defects, androgen insensitivity syndrome, gonadal dysgenesis, 5-alpha reductase deficiency, Klinefelter syndrome, Turner syndrome or PCOS.

Returning to Foucault's legacy, we see that pathologizing the abnormal body is prominently woven throughout the major works of Queer, disability and gender disciplines, and this is particularly true of Judith Butler's work on discourse and gender. Judith Butler's theories, built on but also in conversation with Foucault's later works, have become the compass for contemporary feminist theory. In *Undoing Gender* Butler profiles the contentious debate surrounding a gender identity disorder (GID) diagnosis (later renamed in the Diagnostic and Statistical Manual of Mental Disorders as gender dysphoria). Butler outlines the implications of pathologizing GID and how a diagnosis could affect individual autonomy and access to healthcare resources (*Undoing Gender* 77). This turbulent distinction between normal and pathological comes at a high cost as Butler notes "autonomy is a socially conditioned way of living in the world" (*Undoing Gender* 77). These institutionalized distinctions are far from universally comprehensive as, Butler argues, a GID diagnosis could mean different things for individuals who will fall into these institutionalized categories. For some, the pathologizing of GID could legitimate their health status for access to surgeries, hormonal therapy and insurance coverage. However, being pushed out of the classification of *normal* for other individuals could mean carrying a stigma that there is something deviant about their bodies or gender identity. The reality is that both experiences might be simultaneously true for most.

Butler's perspective on norms and normalization is useful in the work of mapping gender. Butler defines gender as "the apparatus by which the production and normalization of masculine and feminine take place along with the interstitial forms of hormonal, chromosomal, psychic and performative that gender assumes" (*Undoing Gender* 42). Treatments for women with hyperandrogenism which aim to lower "male" hormones directly exemplify these hormonal and performative forms in which gender assumes. Social and medical pressures to present more "feminine" and combat symptoms that are read as "masculine" function as gender regulating as they both produce and normalize the gender binary. Butler suggests that when one exists outside the accepted boundaries of gender, this is a contentious place to be as you are still only discernible in relation to the gender norm. They note, "To be not quite masculine or not quite feminine is still to be understood exclusively in terms of one's relationship to the 'quite masculine' and the 'quite feminine'" (Butler, *Undoing Gender* 42).

This reproduction of the gender binary is evident for women and individuals with hyperandrogenism, and in particular the notion of being "not quite feminine" enough. Some individuals with the disease are held to a standard of femininity that they believe they are not meeting, and in response, some solutions offered by the medical community are to chemically and procedurally alter their bodies until the feminine standard is reached. This dilemma works to inform Butler's understanding of gender as socially produced. They argue that defining gender as existing exclusively on a binary plane of masculine and feminine misses the "critical point" that the ways in which our gender binary is produced are both conditional and come at a significant cost (Butler, *Undoing Gender* 42). I understand Butler's theorizing of gender as an "opening up" of possibilities. They suggest that although there are clear and harmful hegemonic views of gender, variations of gender that are not recognized as normative are "as much a part of gender" as their normative counterparts (Butler, *Undoing Gender* 42). Further, they conclude that although gender is the site of production and normalization of the normative binary of masculine and feminine, gender can also be a place to dismantle and deconstruct these understandings.

From this place of understanding gender as an apparatus of production and normalization, Butler turns to Foucault's theorizing of how discourse works to produce a subject. They conclude that disciplinary discourse not only regulates the subject by making use of them but that it "actively constitutes" the subject (Butler, *Undoing Gender* 50). This process of constituting the subject through disciplinary discourse is evident in the way gender-variant individuals are punished and regulated through both the institutionalized state and through social encounters. Butler offers examples of this including surgical "correction" of "intersexed" individuals, the classification of gender dysphoria disorders including the resulting pathologization, and the state-inflicted regulations on same-sex parents or prospective parents (*Undoing Gender* 55). I would situate the social and medical response to women and individuals with hyperandrogenism within this gendered punishment and regulation as well. The social implications of leaving hyperandrogenous symptoms of excess testosterone "unregulated" are dire and the response from the medical system includes surgical, pharmaceutical and cosmetic interventions. Butler argues that these social and institutional regulations are producing results that remain effectively "unmarked," yet nevertheless, are constituting the boundaries of personhood (*Undoing Gender* 56).

To reinforce their theorizing of gender regulation, Butler engages with the story of David Riemer, a Canadian man who was born a biological male but was raised as a girl following a circumcision procedure that impacted the structure of his penis as an infant. On the advice of a psychologist named John Money, David's parents chose to raise him as a girl named "Brenda" through reassignment surgery and hormones. This decision was made based on Money's theory that gender identity was entirely learned through social reinforcement (Butler, *Undoing Gender* 64). Reportedly, David was never comfortable living as a girl and exhibited behaviour that people in his life understood as stereotypically masculine. After discovering his past at age 14, David chose to return to living life as a male. David's story ultimately became public in 1997 when sexologist Milton Diamond employed David as a case study to ultimately discredit Money's theories on the social constructionism of gender identity. The notable ending to David's story is that he died by suicide in 2004 at the age of 38.

What is most compelling in Butler's analysis of David's story is both the way David's gender was socially and medically regulated and also the ways in which David came to understand and speak about his gender identity. First, Butler notes that the way one's body looks to others constructs the body as gendered (*Undoing Gender* 64). From this place, we may scrutinize medical decisions to perform gender reassignment surgery or hormonal therapy for women and individuals with hyperandrogenism. Butler argues that these procedures are encouraged under the guise of "looking more normal," yet they inflict scars and pain that do not align with this outcome. Butler concludes that gender-variant bodies such as David's (and I would argue some individuals with hyperandrogenism), are "inconceivable" to many and therefore their bodies are regulated through invasive medical practices (*Undoing Gender* 64). Butler stresses that their purpose in employing David's story is not because it proves or disproves either social constructivism or gender essentialism, but rather, they hope to highlight the disciplinary mechanisms used by David to understand and speak about his own gender identity.

This process of self-reporting by David works to unveil the ways in which his gender identity is both affirmed and denied. Because David was subjected to constant unrelenting surveillance, scrutiny and abuse by medical professionals, who collectively dangled gender normalcy just out of reach, he began to understand that he was "failing" gender. The question of whether David was "feminine" enough, or meeting the standard of feminine normalcy, was constantly interrogated. Butler argues that David had come to understand that there was a label of who he should be—stable femininity—and he was not that (*Undoing Gender* 67). This unattainable norm, for David, ensues a certain logic: the norm was distinguishable from the way he felt—it was "other" and therefore he was "other" from stable femininity. Like David, some women and individuals with hyperandrogenism recognize that they too are "failing" femininity. When their bodies express signs of elevated androgens, they experience both external regulation as well as self-regulation in order to resolve this dissonance.

In Butler's chapter entitled "Undiagnosing Gender," they explore the contentious debate surrounding a GID diagnosis and what this diagnosis means for both individual autonomy as well as access to resources. Butler does not attempt to establish an answer to the polarizing GID diagnosis debate but does suggest that autonomy, in different ways, is a socially conditioned way of showing up in the world (*Undoing Gender* 77). In this sense, mechanisms of autonomy, or the opposite such as a GID diagnosis or by extension a hyperandrogenism diagnosis, may be liberating for some and restrictive for others. As Butler points out, those opposing forces usually are occurring simultaneously (*Undoing Gender* 77). Exploring what autonomy might look like for women and individuals with hyperandrogenism seems to reflect Butler's analysis of a GID diagnosis. Some individuals with hyperandrogenism may believe that further reinforcing the condition as a medical illness will legitimize their diagnosis as valid and deserving of healthcare resources including medical research, insurance coverage for medications and the development of pharmaceutical options.

Drawing from their understanding of gender as a site of possibility, Butler contemplates the repercussions of accepting a GID diagnosis as an avenue of autonomy. They wonder what happens to gender as "a mode of becoming" (Butler, *Undoing Gender* 217) when we play within the confines of a masculine/feminine dichotomy. Butler ponders: "Are we stopped in time, made more regular and coherent than we necessarily want to be, when we submit to the norms in order to achieve the entitlements one needs, and the status one desires?" (*Undoing Gender* 81). In conclusion, they rationalize that if a GID diagnosis is facilitating a way in which individuals can achieve their desired autonomy, we have a responsibility to locate a method which cultivates similar effects before we collectively reject a GID rationale (Butler, *Undoing Gender* 82). For women and individuals with hyperandrogenism, I wonder if writing about their illness experience can behave as this "method which cultivates similar effects" Butler is suggesting, these effects including a sense of autonomy.

Butler's discussion of medical practices and the gender norm is particularly useful in understanding hyperandrogenism treatment. Medical procedures and practices that help preserve and foster primary and secondary sex characteristics can include breast augmentation surgery, prescriptions such as Viagra, and, I would argue, hyperandrogenism treatment, including androgen blockers, laser hair removal and topical Rogaine. Butler questions why procedures and treatments that seek to move an individual further away from a gender norm require psychological counselling and interrogation yet practices that position individuals firmly within their gender norm are normalized. Sex becomes culturally understood or readable on the body through these sexed bodily traits. Ultimately, Butler argues that they do not intend to claim that purely cultural signs create a material body, but rather that the body cannot be sexually readable without these signs, which are both inherently cultural and material (*Undoing Gender* 87). Butler is arguing that these processes of being hailed as gendered, or having one's body be sexually readable, function as socially constituted through cultural cues. Although our understandings of gender are established through a combination of cultural and material signifiers, this does not delegitimize gender by rendering it fabricated. In fact, Butler argues, the significance of becoming a gender, and being recognized as such, is vital to one's sense of personhood, one's well-being, and one's ability to "flourish as a bodily being" (*Undoing Gender* 100). Ultimately, Butler calls on nourishing the movement to secure transgender people in positions of medical power as a short-term solution to the GID debate, but ultimately argues for an upheaval of our institutional and cultural understandings of gender norms. This call could reflect an avenue of progress for women and individuals with hyperandrogenism as well.

Through Butler's analysis on GID and "intersex" children, and Foucault's work on sexuality, it is evident that both thinkers have adopted Canguilhem's perspective that the epistemological bases of *normal* and *pathological* are socio-politically constituted. Butler situates gender as a norm to which bodies become regulated. This includes the pathologization of Queerness, disability, GID and "intersex" identities which work to enforce compulsory able-bodiedness and cis-genderness, a perspective adopted by many gender and disability theorists including Robert McRuer, Susannah B. Mintz and

Anne Hunsaker Hawkins. Literature from feminist science studies, "intersex" theory, Queer theory and disability studies can help elucidate the ways that supposedly objective scientific research is in fact part of a larger discursive process that empowers some specific understandings of the body and disempowers others.

Dean Spade and Craig Willse in their 2015 chapter "Norms and Normalization" in *The Oxford Handbook of Feminist Theory*, outline further the legacy of Foucault's work on disciplinary norms for feminist post-structuralism. Spade and Willse argue that Foucault's theorizing of power as productive leaves room for us to consider the mechanisms that allow for the enforcement of norms. The authors suggest, "Bodies, subjectivities, and their relations in space come to be in relation to norms of embodiment, behavior, and thought" (Spade and Willse 553). Ultimately, this discursive conglomerate of power relations yields biopower. In *The History of Sexuality*, Foucault suggests biopower is "an explosion of numerous and diverse techniques for achieving the subjugation of bodies and the control of populations" (140). As Spade and Willse suggest, biopower is actually disciplinary where violent and coercive means of enforcing norms are soon replaced by internalized self-regulation so that "'soft' control replaces direct violence" (554). This understanding of disciplinary power is useful for hyperandrogenism, which complicates and questions assumed biological sex norms. Where I argue that hyperandrogenism unveils the fallacy of the sex binary, there emerges complexity around gender norms and embodiment. For example, we can return to the case study of the Soul Cysters blog, as discussed in the first chapter of this book. For the Soul Cysters, there is a seemingly collective goal to "achieve" normative femininity. It is a convenient conclusion to render the impulse of the Soul Cysters community as disciplinary biopower through self-regulation. However, this leaves "stuff" on the table that has not been engaged with, and that is the matter of the body and the affect of the physical morphing of visible sex characteristics.

It is also significant to note that for hyperandrogenism especially, processes of normalization through regulatory discourse do not suggest that norms are not "real" in the ways that have meaningful impacts on how we organize our sense of identity in relation to the world. This is not to suggest that proponents of regulatory discourse such as Foucault and Butler do not argue this, however. This conclusion leaves space for the political activism and sense of yearning for difference found in gender Queerness. As Spade and Willse suggest, in conversation with Butler's work on GID, mental health diagnoses that centre distress around the failure of gender embodiment or the inability to meet gender norms, work to produce regulatory categories such as "healthy" and "sick" (555). These regulatory discourses have become increasingly insidious in the past several years as social and institutional understandings of transgender identities, for example, have gone from a "sickness" in the brain to a "sickness" in the body. Where diagnosis was centred on attempting to interrogate and cure the distressed mind surrounding gender embodiment, has now shifted to fixing the "wrong" aspects of the sexed body. As Spade and Willse argue, the establishment, preservation and enforcement of these norms are intertwined with systems of scientific expertise, which authorize certain professionals as gatekeepers. This can involve the coercion or denial of medication and other healthcare treatments, including "reparative therapies" and involuntary psychiatric confinement (555). Understanding the complexities of gender and sex difference in relation to identity, as well as the social and institutional oppression of Queer identities, remain essential in reshaping our understanding of health, *sickness*, and the inherent value of diverse identities.

**Colonial Medicine and the Hyperandrogenous Body**

Walking in tandem with the theoretical evolution of the pathologized abnormal body in the context of nuances of biological sex embodiment is the proliferation of colonial medicine. Looking to the work of both Andrea Pitts in her article "White Supremacy, Mass Incarceration, and Clinical Medicine: A Critical Analysis of U.S. Correctional Healthcare" and Mary P. Sutphen and Bridie Andrews in their book entitled *Medicine and Colonial Identity*, colonial medicine may be understood as a nation-building project contingent on gendered and raced practices of conquering and pacifying particular bodies through healthcare resources. Sutphen and Andrews understand colonial medicine as the state ownership over medical knowledge production and knowledge dissemination for the purposes of maintaining hegemonic imperialism. Particularly, the authors argue Western colonial medicine functions as an apparatus of knowledge which works by claiming it holds unknowable truths about the body and pathology (Sutphen and Andrews 15). In this sense, colonial medicine normalizes medical knowledge as exclusively accessible to experts in the healthcare field.

Looking to a historical account of Frantz Fanon's 1959 experiential physician report practicing in French-occupied colonial Algeria, Pitts theorizes colonial medicine as functioning through state ownership over medical knowledge production, as well as the systemic rejection of the racialized patient's subjectivity—or a reducing of the racialized subject to merely a body through the hostile patient/physician encounter ("White Supremacy" 8). In Fanon's experiences as a healthcare provider in mid-century colonial Algeria, white physicians systemically dehumanized Black Algerian patients by giving authority only to what could be visibly seen on the patient's body by delegitimizing any testimonial of lived experience. According to Pitts, the body, then, is assumed to "speak for itself" ("White Supremacy" 8). Black patients' articulation of their subjectivity, including the experience of pain, was routinely positioned as unreliable, disingenuous, or having no grounding in reality by the white physician" (Pitts, "White Supremacy" 8).

Further, Pitts contests, "the experience of illness—the pains, discomforts, longings, and sensations—of the patient are eclipsed...The colonized patient's own lived experience of her/his body becomes irrelevant to the process of forming a medical diagnosis" ("White Supremacy" 8). Pitts concludes by attributing colonial medicine as disinterested in the healthy well-being of the colonial subject, but rather, invested in colonial domination ("White Supremacy" 15). Pitts' discussion of "the politics of knowledge" reinforces this analysis, describing the legacy of colonial medicine as thriving through avenues of state and institutional ownership over knowledge production. Through these strategies, as she names "the politics of knowledge," hegemonic structures are able to maintain control over the production and dissemination of medical information, under the guise of "expertise," which leaves individuals vulnerable to medical coercion—particularly People of Colour (Pitts, "White Supremacy" 8).

In another article entitled "Cruel and Unusual Care and Punishment: Epistemic Injustices in Correctional Health Care," Pitts discusses the idea of hermeneutical injustice, describing it as occurring when a collective lack of understanding unjustly prevents an individual from fully comprehending their own experiences (6). Within a general colonial backdrop, Pitts discusses the kinds of epistemological discourses that emerge as natural truth but are, in fact, rooted in the assimilation, conquering and annihilation of the colonized body. Pitts argues that the history of Indigenous colonization by white settlers has been a history of distorting collective memory where white colonizers have reconfigured Indigenous understanding to believe that they not only relied on the colonizer, but that their "guidance" was necessary for survival ("Cruel and Unusual Care" 8).

Pitts notes that the collective empirical research on race and healthcare exposes a severe gap in the quality of the healthcare experience for People of Colour. Implicating particularly the poor patient/physician encounter, Pitts turns to provider-level factors contributing to the high rates of health disparities among well-meaning white individuals who may not overtly display bias or perceive themselves as prejudiced. She suggests that these individuals may exhibit unconscious stereotyping influenced by overarching attitudes regarding certain beliefs, leading to distorted perceptions at a foundational level (Pitts, "Cruel and Unusual Care" 9). Not only is there a deterioration of the patient/physician encounter that extends to the macro-level to indicate a widespread systematic dysfunction, but also this institutional prejudice is born in the rejection of racial subjectivity. In other words, there exists a systemic reduction of the racialized patient to merely a body void of personal subjectivity. This systemic reduction is reinforced, for example, in cases of pain management.

Studies in clinical medicine find that cases of identical symptoms are often prescribed varying treatments based on the visible racial difference of patients. Physicians systematically rate Black patients lower than white patients on factors such as "intelligence, educational level, level of compliance, likelihood to abuse drugs and alcohol, and likelihood of follow-up with occupational and rehabilitational therapy" (Pitts, "Cruel and Unusual Care" 9). Further, discussing conceptualizations of pain, Pitts offers an example of empirical research that finds male physicians prescribe twice the amount of painkillers to white patients for pain management than Black patients ("Cruel and Unusual Care" 8). Therefore, pain as an embodied experience is neglected in the racialized patient because symptoms of this nature cannot be visually located on the body. Pain of this nature can only be articulated through describing one's own subjective experience and articulations of embodied subjectivity are contingent on believing the patient.

The work of Pitts, Sutphen and Andrews lay the foundation for an understanding of colonial medicine and its implications for Women of Colour today. Research on the experiences of Women of Colour with hyperandrogenism is relatively nonexistent. We know that women with PCOS are at a higher risk than the rest of the population for mental health disorders such as depression, anxiety and body-image distress (Greenwood et al.; Alur-Gupta et al., "Body-Image Distress"). We also know that PCOS affects Women of Colour more frequently and severely than white women (Engmann et al. 493.e1). However, hyperandrogenism does not exist in a vacuum, and its higher prevalence in Women of Colour appears to be connected to the population's higher comorbidity rates. For example, some studies have shown a significantly higher prevalence of metabolic syndrome in Black compared to white women with PCOS (Engmann et al. 493.e1; Hillman et al. 530).

Further, studies have shown that Black women score lower in several PCOS Quality of Life survey domains than white women indicating the lower quality of life (Alur-Gupta et al., "OR25-2 Racial Differences"). Most of the research on Indigenous women with hyperandrogenism is brief, does not refer to women's experiences, and typically discusses PCOS in relation to the higher relevance of diabetes in Indigenous populations. For example, Wilson et al. discuss in their article "First Nations, Inuit, and Métis Women's Sexual and Reproductive Health" that Indigenous women have an increased prevalence of obesity due to a shift towards a more sedentary lifestyle, coupled with greater food insecurity and limited access to recreational facilities faced by many Indigenous women. This prevalence could lead to higher rates of PCOS/metabolic syndrome, which, in turn, may negatively affect their fertility (S31). There is a critical need to research the experiences of Women of Colour who have hyperandrogenism to better understand the effects of the disease on mental and physical health.

**Uncanny Hyperandrogenism and the Need to Tell Our Story**

The extremely muddy terrain of the path in which hyperandrogenous bodies become destabilized and take form within and outside of the normal, pathological and colonial discursive currents discussed above, has been on my mind for years. In an article I published in *The Canadian Review of Comparative Literature* called "Illness of the Gendered Body, Freud's *The Uncanny*, and 'Being-in-the-World,'" I argue that the phenomenological experience of sex-based illness can be understood through a theoretical framework of both Sigmund Freud's *The Uncanny* as well as Heidegger's notion of an unhomelike being-in-the-world (Perram, "Illness of the Gendered Body" 592). This article turns to the work of phenomenologist Fredrik Svenaeus who has laid the theoretical foundation for connecting *The Uncanny* to the experience of illness, most notably in his case study of anorexia nervosa.

I argue, in this work, that the phenomenological experience of sex-based illnesses such as hyperandrogenism mirrors *The Uncanny* by distorting temporal reality by making alien both the past and future, rendering the body and therefore identity and selfhood abnormal, and finally working to trouble the notion of the everyday (Perram, "Illness of the Gendered Body" 592). First, a hyperandrogenous body poses the threat of "morphing" into the alien unfamiliar where suddenly one's understanding of their identity in relation to the past and future is challenged. I note

> With hyperandrogenism, the destabilization of subjecthood is twofold. Supplementing the otherness of our human body, another layer—the gendered body—ties together sociocultural, historical, and political framing of biological sex, bodily appearance, and behaviour. We are not only bodies but gendered bodies.
>
> (Perram, "Illness of the Gendered Body" 594)

Ultimately, when our understanding of health is tied to cultural notions of normative, binary sex expression, a distortion of the body across sexed lines forces one to relinquish their sense of identity. Further, temporally, hyperandrogenism disrupts our notion of the ordinary everyday, or our sense of "being-in-the-world." The illness reveals to you that you are no longer in the realm of normalcy but are, in fact, in a subversive reality where you now must try to escape and "return" to the everyday. From here, hyperandrogenism may disrupt first our sense of identity, and second our sense of temporality. Once illness has made our body alien to our self, "A crack splits through the temporal narrative of the self, igniting a need to rewrite the identity of the past in order to preserve the identity of the future" (Perram, "Illness of the Gendered Body" 598). In this sense, there becomes a need to reconstruct our story in ways that keep our identities and sense of temporality intact.

When this scramble to keep the identity intact feels like water through the hands, some authors turn to illness narratives in order to write their bodies into a budding biopolitics. What can be learned from turning to hypertext illness narratives as an avenue to theoretically explore both the complexity of gendered subjectivity and the cultural construction of illness? Perhaps by turning to autobiographical accounts, we may locate the interface between the construction of the gendered self and what we may consider biogenetic dysfunction. In her 1993 autobiographical account of her medical subjugation with breast cancer, "Queer and Now," Eve Kosofsky Sedgwick reflects that "being a breast cancer patient [...] plunges one into an experience of almost archetypal Femaleness" (13). The experience of breast cancer heightens, for Sedgwick, an astute awareness of the gendered cultural constructions that come into contact with her body, and frankly, always have. Sedgwick witnesses the deep medical and social attention paid to her breasts—scrutiny over their shape, size, *sickness*, presence and absence—which unveils a truth about gendered embodiment. This truth is that our cultural, institutional and belief systems are hardwired to understand and maintain a prescriptive gendered body. To extrapolate from this, I wonder, how are experiences of hyperandrogenism, for some, hailed into larger narratives of hegemonic femininity? At the core of this book is a drive to understand how these contemplations take form in the stories of the *Click Me* authors.

## Works Cited

Alur-Gupta, Snigdha, et al. "Body-Image Distress Is Increased in Women with Polycystic Ovary Syndrome and Mediates Depression and Anxiety." *Fertility Sterility*, vol. 112, no. 5, 2019a, pp. 930–938.e1.

Alur-Gupta, Snigdha, et al. "OR25-2 Racial Differences in Anxiety, Depression, and Quality of Life Between White and Black Women with PCOS and Controls." *Journal of the Endocrine Society*, vol. 3, no.1, 2019b. Online Print.

The Associated Press. "Track Officials Called Caster Semenya 'Biologically Male,' Newly Released Documents Show." *The New York Times*, 18 June 2019, https://www.nytimes.com/2019/06/18/sports/track-officials-called-caster-semenya-biologically-male-newly-released-documents-show.html.

Badawy, Ahmed, and Abubaker Elnashar. "Treatment Options for Polycystic Ovary Syndrome." *International Journal of Women's Health*, vol. 3, 2011, pp. 25–35.

Basile, Lisa Marie. "Why PCOS Affects Women of Color Differently." *Endocrine Web*, 13 November 2020, https://www.endocrineweb.com/news/polycystic-ovary-syndrome-pcos/63344-why-pcos-affects-women-color-differently. Accessed 1 March 2021.

Butler, Judith. *Bodies That Matter: On the Discursive Limits of "Sex"*. Routledge, 2011.

Butler, Judith. *Undoing Gender*. Routledge, 2004, pp. 40–56.

Canguilhem, Georges. *The Normal and the Pathological*. Zone Books, 1991.

Cannon, Brandy. *Diagnosis and Management of Polycystic Ovary Syndrome: A Literature Review*. Pacific University, PhD Dissertation, 2008.

Cooky, Cheryl and Shari L. Dworkin. "Policing the Boundaries of Sex: A Critical Examination of Gender Verification and the Caster Semenya Controversy." *The Journal of Sex Research*, vol. 50, no. 2, 2013, pp. 103–111.

Ekback, Maria, et al. "It Is Always on My Mind": Women's Experiences of Their Bodies When Living with Hirsutism." *Health Care for Women International*, vol. 30, no. 5, 2009, pp. 358–372.

Engmann, Lawrence, et al. "Racial and Ethnic Differences in the Polycystic Ovary Syndrome (PCOS) Metabolic Phenotype." *American Journal of Obstetrics and Gynecology*, vol. 216, no. 5, 2017, pp. 493.e1–493.e13.

Fausto-Sterling, Anne. "The Five Sexes: Why Male and Female Are Not Enough." *Sciences*, vol. 33, 1993, pp. 20–20.

Findlay, Deborah. "Discovering Sex: Medical Science, Feminism and Intersexuality." *Canadian Review of Sociology/Revue Canadienne de Sociologie*, vol. 32, no. 1, 2008, pp. 25–52.

Foucault, Michel. *Discipline and Punish*. Penguin, 1991.

Foucault, Michel. *The History of Sexuality, Vol. II: The Use of Pleasure*. Translated by Robert Hurley, Penguin, 1985.

Galic, Isabel, et al. "Disparities in Access to Fertility Care: Who's In and Who's Out." *F&S Reports*, vol. 2, no. 1, 2021, pp. 109–117.

Gibson-Helm, Melanie, et al. "Delayed Diagnosis and a Lack of Information Associated with Dissatisfaction in Women with Polycystic Ovary Syndrome." *The Journal of Clinical Endocrinology & Metabolism*, vol. 102, no. 2, 2017, pp. 604–612,

Goodley, Dan. *Disability Studies: An Interdisciplinary Introduction*. Sage, 2011.

Greenwood, Eleni A., et al. "Depression Over the Lifespan in a Population-Based Cohort of Women with Polycystic Ovary Syndrome: Longitudinal Analysis." *The Journal of Clinical Endocrinology & Metabolism*, vol. 104, no. 7, 2019, pp. 2809–2819.

Hillman Jennifer K., et al. "Black Women with Polycystic Ovary Syndrome (PCOS) have Increased Risk for Metabolic Syndrome and Cardiovascular Disease Compared with White Women with PCOS." *Fertility and Sterility*, vol. 101, no. 2, 2014, pp. 530–535.

Himelein, Melissa J., and Samuel S. Thatcher. "Depression and Body Image Among Women with Polycystic Ovary Syndrome." *Journal of Health Psychology*, vol. 11, no. 4, 2006, pp. 613–625.

Hoyos, Luis R., et al. "Measures of Patient Dissatisfaction with Health Care in Polycystic Ovary Syndrome: Retrospective Analysis." *Journal of Medical Internet Research*, vol. 22, no. 4, 2020, e16541.

Ingle, Sean. "Semenya Loses Landmark Legal Case Against IAAF Over Testosterone Levels." *The Guardian*, 1 May 2019. Archived from the original on 30 March 2023. Retrieved 28 October 2023.

Kristeva, Julia. *Powers of Horror: An Essay on Abjection*. Columbia University Press, 1982.

Lucidi, Richard Scott, Ed. "Polycystic Ovarian Syndrome Clinical Presentation." *Medscape*, 2016.

Magubane, Zine. "Spectacles and Scholarship: Caster Semenya, Intersex Studies, and the Problem of Race in Feminist Theory." *Signs*, vol. 39, no. 3, 2014, pp. 761–785.

*Medscape*. WebMD LLC, 1992, https://www.medscape.com/.

Mather, Victor, and Jeré Longman. "Ruling Leaves Caster Semenya with Few Good Options." *The New York Times*, 31 July 2019. Archived from the original on 18 November 2023. Retrieved 19 August 2019.

Perram, Megan. "Illness of the Gendered Body, Freud's *The Uncanny*, and 'being-in-the-world'." *Canadian Review of Comparative Literature*, vol. 46, no. 4, 2019, pp. 587–600.

Pfister, Gertrude, and Kristine Rømer. "'It's Not Very Feminine to Have a Mustache': Experiences of Danish Women with Polycystic Ovary Syndrome." *Health Care for Women International*, vol. 38, no. 2, 2017, pp. 167–186.

Pitts, Andrea. "Cruel and Unusual Care and Punishment: Epistemic Injustices in Correctional Health Care." *APA Newsletters*, vol. 14, no. 1, 2014, pp. 6–9.

Pitts, Andrea. "White Supremacy, Mass Incarceration, and Clinical Medicine: A Critical Analysis of U.S. Correctional Healthcare." *Radical Philosophy Review (Philosophy Documentation Center)*, vol. 18, no. 2, 2015, pp. 267–285.

Rachoń, D. "Differential Diagnosis of Hyperandrogenism in Women with Polycystic Ovary Syndrome." *Experimental and Clinical Endocrinology & Diabetes*, vol. 120, no. 4, 2012, pp. 205–209.

Sedgwick, Eve Kosofsky. "Queer and Now." *Tendencies*, 1993, pp. 1–20.

"Semenya Case Referred to European Rights Court's Grand Chamber." *Reuters*, 6 November 2023. Archived from the original on 12 November 2023. Retrieved 19 March 2024.

Semenya, Caster. "Running in a Body That's My Own." *The New York Times*, 21 October 2023. Archived from the original on 28 October 2023. Retrieved 28 October 2023.

Sonksen, Peter, et al. "Medical and Ethical Concerns Regarding Women with Hyperandrogenism and Elite Sport." *The Journal of Clinical Endocrinology & Metabolism*, vol. 100, no. 3, 2015, pp. 825–827.

*Soul Cysters Dot Net*. vBulletin Solutions, Inc., 2022, https://www.soulcysters.net/.

Spade, Dean, and Criag Willse. "Norms and Normalization." *The Oxford Handbook of Feminist Theory*, edited by Lisa Disch and Mary Hawkesworth, Oxford University Press, 2015.

Spary, Sara. "Caster Semenya Appeals to European Court of Human Rights Over 'Discriminatory' Testosterone Limit." *CNN*, 26 February 2021. Archived from the original on 9 October 2023. Retrieved 22 March 2021.

Sutphen, Mary P., and Bridie Andrews. *Medicine and Colonial Identity*. Routledge, 2003.

Svenaeus, Fredrik. "Anorexia Nervosa and the Body Uncanny: A Phenomenological Approach." *Philosophy, Psychiatry, and Psychology*, vol. 20, no. 1, 2013, pp. 81–91.

Svenaeus, Fredrik. *Phenomenological Bioethics: Medical Technologies, Human Suffering, and the Meaning of Being Alive*. Routledge, 2018.

Svenaeus, Fredrik. "The Body Uncanny–Further Steps Towards a Phenomenology of Illness." *Medicine, Health Care and Philosophy*, vol 3, 2000, pp. 125–137.

Wilson, Don, et al. "First Nations, Inuit, and Métis Women's Sexual and Reproductive Health." *Journal of Obstetrics and Gynaecology Canada*, vol. 35, no. 6, 2013, pp. S28–S32.

Wu, Diane. "The Unnecessary Use of Gender Verification in Sport." Queen's University, J.D. Candidate, June 2019.

Yoo, Richard Y., et al. "Questionnaire on Self-Perception and Behavior of Adolescent Girls with Polycystic Ovary Syndrome (PCOS)." *Fertility & Sterility*, vol. 80, no. 3, 2003, p. 3.

# 3 Digital Messengers

## Hypertext

### Feminist New Materialism and Digital Materiality

I first encountered the term feminist new materialism back in 2016 during my time in graduate school pursuing my master's degree. I was taking a course on prison abolitionism, when a classmate was looking into the concept for a paper. They were using feminist new materialism as a theoretical framework to analyze the experiences of incarcerated mothers and pregnant women. If memory serves me, feminist new materialism provided them with a productive lens through which to grapple with the sensory impact of giving birth behind bars. While the topic was intriguing, I found myself hesitant to look deeper into feminist new materialism. At the time, I struggled to grasp its concepts fully, perceiving them as too abstract and slippery to offer any practical value to my work. Content with my Foucauldian frameworks and poststructuralist theories, I avoided any further engagement with feminist new materialism throughout the remainder of that degree. However, it was not long before I found myself revisiting it, waist-deep in the writing process of my dissertation literature review a few years later.

The literature review is truly a Goliath. Finding an effective method to triage and consolidate the development of multiple theories over the course of time takes organization, to say the least. In the process of writing my literature review chapter of my dissertation, I came to understand literature reviews as methodological endeavours that actively produce connections. These connections ultimately form the foundation for a specific theoretical framework and provide justification for the chosen methodological approach in a research project. A well-executed literature review should assemble a relational network of the topic, coming to a crux right where the research question begins. In essence, if you have done your literature review right, your theoretical framework reveals itself at the intersection of all the theories and perspectives that have shaped your topic up to that point. I suppose I must have done my literature review correctly, because it eventually led me back to feminist new materialism.

DOI: 10.4324/9781003646921-3

Feminist new materialism is an expansive field of study that comes out of feminist science studies, environmental humanities, Queer and affect theory, and, notably, the legacy of Gilles Deleuze and Félix Guattari's *A Thousand Plateaus*. Feminist new materialism works with theories of the posthuman body in relation to ontology to see beyond a focus on language and discourse to invite in a more materialist-embodied understanding of the world. According to scholar Sarah E. Truman, feminist new materialism can be regarded as both a theoretical framework and a methodological approach, with the latter advocating for the direct implication of researchers in qualitative research, the challenging of positivism, and the re-centring of non- and more-than-human agents (2). Feminist new materialism has become a grounding contact point for the work of this book because it offers a novel toolkit to think about hyperandrogenism and digital illness narratives. Aspects of this toolkit will be explored in depth below, however, here, I must bring to the forefront the critical notion of feminism in feminist new materialism. This framework holds a kinship with feminism as a method of centring the diverse experiences of marginalized identities. This is significant, as Truman argues, because feminist new materialism engages in conversation with an array of fields including physics, science and mathematics to explore the role of "more-than-human" agents (2). Foregrounding feminism in this work is an ongoing project to mitigate the risk of reproducing a normative (white, male, cis, able-bodied and straight) subject.

Feminist new materialism, ultimately, is a diverse discipline with contractions, inconsistencies, and divergence within the perspectives of its proponents. However, the foundational beliefs of feminist new materialism form in a community of scholars that are attuned to exploring materiality and more-than-human subject formation. Notable scholars who have shaped the field include Karen Barad, Donna Haraway, Anne Marie Balsamo, Sadie Plant, Rosi Braidotti, Myra J. Hird, Jasbir Puar, Patricia Clough and Victoria Pitts-Taylor in their collective works in feminist science studies, cyborg theory, gender and cultural studies, and affect theory. Feminist new materialism is in response to the "extra-discursive" perspectives on subject formation and calls for consideration of how matter comes to inform discursive experience. According to Kameron Sanzo in their 2018 article entitled "New Materialism(s)," the discourses associated with new materialism(s) align with posthumanism by aiming to redefine the human within a framework that includes nonhuman actors. These discourses challenge the notion of a stable, individualistic, liberal subject and advocate for a critical materialist examination of the worldwide, interconnected impacts of late capitalism and climate change (para. 1). What drew me to feminist new materialism theory is its turn to matter as a deeply vital reality. There is something important that the materiality of the body brings to our narratives and this book questions what that materiality means and how it goes on to shape both experience and discourse.

The field of feminist new materialism brings together a collective challenging of the seeming omnipotence of the linguistic turn that has dominated academia for decades and a call for both a decentring of humanism and a turn to affective materiality. Feminist new materialism responds to humanistic perspectives of a Cartesian mind–body split and the ways in which this binary evokes similar binaries in response, including nature–culture, human–animal and subject–object. This rejection of binary formations, for feminist new materialists, calls into question the ways in which the matter of "objects" has been taken up as passive. Vitality is a term employed heavily in the feminist new materialism theoretical movement, which speaks to matter's agency through its ability to enact relational affect on other forms of matter. As Truman notes, if agency and vitality are not exclusive to humans but instead inherent in all matter, it forces us to contend with notions of causality, existence, the interaction of phenomena and ultimately, responsibility. This positionality requires a rethinking of the politics of collaboration and research ethics, where we must acknowledge that nonhuman entities, too, possess agency. This agency, then, challenges traditional views on how we approach cooperation and ethical practices in research (Truman 4). The concept of the "new" inherent in feminist new materialism, according to Truman, is in response to a psychoanalytic form of Marxism that positions culture, politics and history as material struggles rather than older perspectives of materialism which reified phenomena in human agency (2). Feminist new materialism turns "back" to materialism in a novel way that does not start with a historical conceptualization, but rather, affective matter. Here is where the distinction between old and new materialism emerges. Truman notes, however, these frameworks should not be approached as in opposition to each other but working with both the "liveliness" of matter and the politics of subject formation.

Feminist new materialism has emerged in response to the dominant philosophies of the linguistic turn, which was inclusive of both structuralism and poststructuralism. As shown in Chapter 2, the research of this book draws heavily from theories that dominated poststructuralism, specifically theory on "intersex" bodies. At first, these discourse-heavy theories appear to be incongruent with feminist new materialism as a theoretical framework that emerged in response to the language-focused linguistic turn. Following further reading into feminist new materialism as an expansive movement, I now understand that although feminist new materialism is critical of poststructuralist dominance, I do not believe them to be mutually exclusive. In fact, the ways I employ feminist new materialism in this project about "intersex" bodies truly benefit from building off of poststructuralist beliefs rather than rejecting them outright. This is because poststructuralism offers ways to understand the discursively constructed aspects of biological sex, whereas feminist new materialism centres the materiality of the body in relation to technology. Truman parallels this argument that the linguistic and material turns can work in relation to each other. Scholars of feminist new materialism have been misattributed to calling for an end to language as a significant entity of research, however, many proponents of feminist new materialism understand that language and discourse are material things.

Scholars such as Fausto-Sterling have adopted a feminist new materialism stance by emphasizing the deeply penetrable bodily difference of subjects, including the ways in which our cells react differently in varying environmental contexts (Sanzo). Identity and difference are, as Sanzo suggests, outputs of the ways in which matter intersects with bodies and the larger social and environmental spaces in which bodies inhabit. Feminist new materialism looks to the affective turn to counter the seeming limitations of the linguistic turn's exclusive affinity to subject formation through discourse. Affect theory considers the relationality of bodies through unconscious means. Through the work of Baruch Spinoza, affect has come to be understood by theorists as "the capacities of bodies to act or be acted upon by other bodies" (Truman 5). Affect theory holds roots in Deleuzian ontology and argues that, unlike emotion, affect is a pre-personal experience that lays the foundations for, but is independent of, signification, language, and representation. As Truman argues, affective capacities are produced through relational tugs from "intensities, proximities and viscosities" that swirl inside, between, across, and even "stick to" certain bodies (4). According to Truman, theories that incorporate affect tend to pay attention to how bodies relate and become rather than how bodies are. Some interpretations of affect theory that centre a pre-discursive moment have, however, been challenged by Queer, feminist and critical disability scholars who argue that this perspective runs the risk of delegitimizing the affect of political forms of identity formation (Truman 4). Therefore, these scholars have prioritized finding ways to understand affect in relation to intersectionality. Assemblage theory emerged from this vantage point.

Through terms such as *assemblages* and *rhizomes*, feminist new materialism is concerned with the relationality between parts. In 2007, Karen Barad wrote *Meeting the Universe Halfway: Quantum Physics and the Entanglement of Matter and Meaning* where they put forward the concept of intra-action in response to interaction. Barad argues that intra-action is a signifier for mutually constituted agents that are in an entanglement with each other (*Meeting the Universe Halfway* 33). Truman argues that the term "interaction" is faulty as it presupposes the existence of distinct, individualized agents prior to the interaction. In contrast, "intra-action" conceptualizes phenomena as specific material configurations involving humans, nonhumans, animals and materials that do not exist independently of their relationality (4). What is significant for understanding the experience of hyperandrogenism, in response to the concept of intra-action, is adopting Barad's claim that as a researcher, you are always already entangled in the process and outcomes of your research. Even through the act of observation you are actively intra-acting with and affecting other bodies of matter and this must be taken into account. Ultimately, for Barad, this means a way of contending with the world while simultaneously being a part of it (*Meeting the Universe Halfway* 88). This concept of intra-action of the researcher with the research is vital for the *Click Me* research because I am questioning the material realities of women and nonbinary individuals with hyperandrogenism, specifically how the body comes to interact with the digital-material, however, I understand it is critical to implicate myself in this analysis. Mainly, I wonder how I come to affect the data generated. How does my lived experience with hyperandrogenism come to shape the outcome of this research and the experiences of the *Click Me* authors?

## Assemblage Theory or "What Is It Like to Feel Hair Growing on the Surface of the Face?"

In their book *A Thousand Plateaus*, Gilles Deleuze and Félix Guattari develop the ontological framework of assemblage theory. This theory argues that the "parts" that make-up the whole of a body are not fixed, but rather, fluid, exchangeable and entangled with "parts" of external bodies. Assemblage theory plays with assumptions of scale. For example, the theory challenges notions that "wholes" are singular, organic or "pure" entities. Rather, "wholes" are made-up of individualized "parts" which intra-act with other, external "wholes." Assemblage theory came out of Deleuze and Guattari's work on dynamical systems theory which looks at how systems of material organize themselves. The scholars adapted this theory to include not only the material but also linguistic, social and philosophical elements, to produce assemblage theory. Deleuze and Guattari use three intra-acting terms to work with the concept of assemblage: coding, stratification and territorialization. These terms vary but are reliant on each other to function.

As Daniel Smith and John Protevi explain in *The Stanford Encyclopedia of Philosophy*,

> Coding is the process of ordering matter as it is drawn into a body; by contrast, stratification is the process of creating hierarchical bodies, while territorialization is the ordering of those bodies in 'assemblages,' that is to say, an emergent unity joining together heterogeneous bodies in a 'consistency.'

Deleuze and Guattari evoke the analogy of the constellation to explore these terms. A constellation is composed of an imaginative rendering that relies on the organization of matter in a particular order to create a body. This process of ordering to render the imaginative "reality" of the constellation is called coding. From here, Deleuze and Guattari argue that some "heavenly bodies" are included in our imagining of the constellation, and some are left out. This is dependent on where the stars are located, how close together they are, and how well they serve the larger project of rendering the constellation. This process of hierarchizing various bodies to form a territory is called stratification (Smith and Protevi). Territorialization, the final concept that completes the triad, is the process of organizing bodies in ways that create the larger assemblage. The process of territorialization can be of material bodies, such as humans and more-than-humans, or bodies of signification. Further, processes of deterritorialization and reterritorialization explore the ways in which parts become disconnected or reconnected to the larger body.

The conceptualization of Deleuze and Guattari's notion of assemblage theory is highly complex. It has been taken up in a myriad of disciplines including philosophy, political science, and, significant for this research, feminist new materialism. In 2012, Jasbir K. Puar wrote the article "'I Would Rather be a Cyborg than a Goddess': Becoming-Intersectional in Assemblage Theory" which explores the use of assemblage theory through feminist new materialism and as a response to theories of intersectionality. For Puar, assemblages are important because, first, these perspectives challenge the traditional view of the human body as a distinct, organic entity. According to Haraway, the body extends beyond its physical boundaries, leaving traces of DNA everywhere and containing other bodies within, such as microbes and bacteria. Humans are interconnected with various forces, affects and energies, forming composite entities of information. Second, assemblages reject the privileging of human bodies and transcend the human/animal binary. In addition to de-emphasizing the uniqueness of human bodies, they recognize that various forms of matter can constitute bodies, including water, cities and institutions. Matter is considered an active agent in these perspectives (Puar 380). This is a critical understanding of assemblages for hyperandrogenism because it allows a shift in the conversation away from discussions of norms and performativity (which are important but dominant), to discussions about the biological mechanisms of the body. It allows us to ask questions such as: what is it like to feel hair growing on the surface of the face? What and how are bodily receptors *receiving* with the body's influx of pharmaceuticals? It also allows us to explore the ways in which the body intersects with hypertext technology in the process of narrative writing.

Most significant for hyperandrogenism that assemblage theory offers is a way into a critical understanding of identity. The participant make-up of the

*Click Me* project was diverse[1] and issues of race, sexuality, gender identity and ability must be accounted for. I spent a lot of time with the theory on feminist new materialism thinking about intersectionality—a framework I was originally intending to work with—and the ways in which it could offer tools to pay attention to identity politics in this work. The more research I was able to do, however, the more insight I found on employing assemblage theory over intersectionality. Puar argues that intersectionality has come to be understood as the first-line-approach for feminist theorizing of difference for the past thirty years.

Intersectionality, a concept developed by Kimberlé Crenshaw in 1989, emerged from second-wave Black feminist thought that was challenging white-centric modes of approaching critical theory. Notably, Crenshaw used the analogy of the intersection of a traffic stop to explain how aspects of an individual's social and political identities, such as gender identity, class, sex, race, sexuality and ability, intersect to create different modes of discrimination and privilege. Intersectionality, however, recently has been challenged by some scholars due to the framework's seeming reification of a standard, "neutral" identity in which all others become variants (Puar 371). Puar argues that, as presented by transnational, postcolonial and critical race theorists, the positioning of white women at the centre of subjecthood has been reasserted through the deployment of intersectionality (373). Puar, then, calls for a Queer assemblage framework to supplement the short-comings of intersectionality, as not oppositional but "frictional" to each other (372). Feminist scholars of new materialism, such as Donna Haraway, Elizabeth Grosz and Karan Barad, have argued that intersectionality is a "gridlock model" (Puar 56) that fails to embody the structures to account for nonrepresentational matter as unstable assemblages that cannot be easily pulled apart into distinct identity formations. In Donna Haraway's prolific 1985 essay "A Cyborg Manifesto: Science, Technology, and Socialist-Feminism in the Late Twentieth Century," she concludes her analysis by proclaiming that she would rather be a cyborg than a goddess. This analogy, according to Puar, is Haraway's claiming of a postmodern more-than-human body by rejecting the historized and racialized body, which produces a distinction between assemblages and intersectionality (57). Many scholars have challenged Haraway's use of a racialized monarch to foil the posthuman body, suggesting that a declaration of desiring the posthuman body is an avoidance of theorizing race relations.

Puar argues that this is a significant critique, however, it bypasses that linguistic performativity assumes that all meaning is confined to language (58). Ultimately, the distinctions between intersectionality and assemblage theory are rooted in a divergence in the conceptualization of identity. For intersectionality, experience is produced through the intersection of multiple identity parts in the subject. These identities can be "pulled out" and analyzed in how they relate to the sociopolitical experience. Assemblages, on the other hand, allow for the evolution, subtraction and addition of identities. These identities cannot be "pulled out" to examine their relationships, nor do they hold individualized meaning. Unlike intersectionality, meaning is found in the assemblage. Ultimately, my choice for turning to assemblage theory over intersectionality is critical for the *Click Me* research because it affords a way to conceive of agency. Where intersectionality might view identity as a collection of predetermined parts that everyone is a combination of, assemblages account for "things" outside the body to compose identity.

In 2004, N. Katherine Hayles published "Print is Flat, Code is Deep: The importance of media-specific analysis," a crucial work in hypertext theory. Hayles emphasizes the need for scholars to view text as an embodied material entity, which is a dynamic quality arising from the interaction between the text as a physical artefact, its conceptual content and the interpretive activities of readers and writers. She argues against the notion that texts are immaterial, highlighting the differences between text on screen and text in print. Hayles' work is foundational because it introduces feminist new materialism into hypertext theory and it addresses the complexities of text production politics. Hayles believes that the materiality of hypertext involves the interactive meaning-making processes between the physical aspects and the language's signification. These meaning-making processes take form in later chapters of this book, but involve the relationality between code, hormones, hair, flesh, identity and, critically, hypertext.

## Matter and Hypertext

Are you still here? While the above trek through the theoretical underpinnings of feminist new materialism is dense, I believe it is important to lay the foundation for how matter comes to matter in this book. It was helpful, in the analysis of the *Click Me* research, to engage with feminist new materialism concepts in ways that first, ironically, deconstructed the theory into parts. I started by asking: what is inherently feminist about feminist new materialism? Rebecca Coleman, Tara Page and Helen Palmer argue in "Feminist New Materialist Practice: The Mattering of Methods" that the feminism of feminist new materialism is embodied in an approach to challenging power relations in non-dualistic and potentially generative ways. The authors argue that the labour required to delegitimize conventional, abstract reasoning in order to legitimize the "messy mattering of methods" is the same energy required for dismantling structures of oppression that position different as less than. This energy, according to the authors, is feminist energy concerned with not only concepts, but bodies, ontologies, nature and biology. The ways in which the *Click Me* data was analyzed,[2] for example, was attuned to the feminism inherent in feminist new materialism. In particular, I positioned myself, as the researcher, to question how I have acted responsibly in conducting this research. Responsibility, in this context, is described as actively benefiting marginalized humans and more-than-humans in its affect. This affect may look like networks that become generated, various relations or worlds built in the wake of the research.

This need for responsibility, I believe, was met in the *Click Me* research in several ways. Most notably the outcomes of the research, discussed in Chapter 6, aim to contribute a resource for marginalized individuals to respond to illness. But I also grappled with this responsibility through my relationship with the *Click Me* authors. Sarah. E. Truman's approach to qualitative research, adopted in this project, argues that feminist new materialism approaches to research should be concerned with implicating the researcher in the process of data analysis (2). I am a researcher who also lives with the disease I am studying. I share similar experiences with the *Click Me* authors and can empathize with their stories. This is a truth that will inevitably affect research outcomes and the interpretation of the data. However, rather than resisting my implication, I chose to make it an intentional aspect of my feminist research design. This feminist new materialism approach is reflexive because the story of the author is situated within the context of their lifeworld, and mine as well. An important element of this method is that the influence of the researcher's subjectivity and lifeworld is both inevitable and a valuable contribution to the analysis. In this feminist new materialism framework, the researcher's implication is seen as not only vital but always already entangled within the research.

I made an effort in every author encounter to find moments to articulate aspects of my own story or to note, when appropriate, that I had experienced something similar to what an author was sharing. My mark on the research and the outcomes of the research is present, even if I had not chosen to actively share my own illness experience with the *Click Me* authors. This choice to do so, though, was an attempt to embrace the implication in the open. These efforts were later represented in the code "Researcher Implication," as depicted in Chapter 5, Table 5.1. The strategy I took in both screening and closing interviews was to contribute snippets of my own illness experience in an authentic way. These moments typically involved responding with empathy to an author's descriptions of a dehumanizing experience in the healthcare system or with their illness in general and echoing that sentiment through my own personal experience. For example, in response to an author revealing feelings of subjugation following a doctor's appointment, I responded:

> I think the common experience that I'm hearing amongst my participants, and also my own experience with PCOS, in the healthcare system, has been, like, extremely dehumanizing. Not all the time, but like these, like microaggressions, I guess, like, these small encounters that really just are dehumanizing, right?

In other moments, I chose to affirm, through personal experience, statements made by authors who discussed the benefits of writing about their illness. For example, to one author I explained:

> That's, that's amazing because that's exactly how I feel. I think it's so like, helpful to tell your story. But I have a hard time like talking out loud about what I'm going through with people because it's just like, kind of awkward, right? But when I write about it, I find it so much better. And especially if it's anonymous, because then it's just like your name isn't on it. You can actually just really like get everything out there.[3]

Ultimately, the feminist foundations of feminist new materialism were a sentiment I actively tried to foreground in the ways in which I carried out and analysed the *Click Me* research. I believe this approach harkens back to Coleman et al.'s description of a mirrored energy between feminism and new materialism. This energy, in both cases, is concerned with deconstructing barriers and binaries and embracing difference. For this book, this energy also includes challenging traditional belief systems around the removed researcher yielding unbiased results. The research is a tangled myriad of agents: authors, the Twine software, memory, stories, bodies, symptoms, etc. And I am in this mess, too.

The second question I considered in my approach to a feminist new materialism methodology was: how am I centring matter in this research? Coleman et al. argue that a key tenet of new materialist thought is the understanding that "matter" is inherently multiple, self-organizing, dynamic and inventive, and, through this lens, operates across the boundaries of nature and culture, the animate and the inanimate, as well as between bodies and environments. Materiality, then, is embodied entanglement of a multitude of matter. The authors argue that academia has resisted the simple uptake of the mattering of matter through sensory perception. For the authors sensory perception is a critical component for contending with material thinking and practice (Coleman et al.). To centre matter in the *Click Me* research came down to designing the writing prompt of the literary hypertext illness narrative in a way that called on authors to explore sensory embodiment.

The free writing storyboard prompt asked: "In this Moment, how did it feel to be in your body? What do you see, smell, taste, or hear?" The final writing prompt for the hypertext illness narratives strategically builds on the previous question to ask: "What is it like to live in a body with hyperandrogenism?" The prompts in the *Click Me* module intentionally call on authors to centre their embodied, rather than conceptual, experience of the disease and to think about how illness feels growing into the body.

The framing of these writing prompts situated matter in the authors' stories in ways that may not have been captured otherwise. Table 5.1, in Chapter 5, shows that during analysis, the concept "Matter" was coded 20 times throughout the corpus of the *Click Me* research. What constituted as matter in the stories was informed by Rosi Braidotti's concept of neo-materialism as "a method, a conceptual frame and a political stand, which refuses the linguistic paradigm, stressing instead the concrete yet complex materiality of bodies immersed in social relations of power" (Dolphijn and van der Tuin 21). Like all concepts, the practice of coding this concept was highly mediated by my interpretation. It did, however, pinpoint compelling references to how the hyperandrogenous body becomes a relational force within power dynamics. For example, one *Click Me* author explores how their disease feels like the prickly sensation of coarse hair growing from their chin. Another author, as shown in Figure 3.1, wrote: "The hot wax feels like it burns as its spread thin across my face. Without warning, it is soon ripped off, occassionally [sic] taking bits of the top layer of skin with it due to carelessness." In this research, this is how matter is centred—through the embodied interactions between body parts, wax, technology, code, stubble and hypertext.

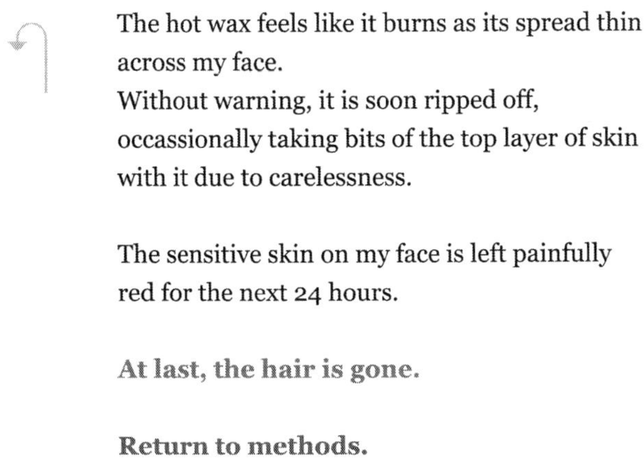
The hot wax feels like it burns as its spread thin
across my face.
Without warning, it is soon ripped off,
occassionally taking bits of the top layer of skin
with it due to carelessness.

The sensitive skin on my face is left painfully
red for the next 24 hours.

**At last, the hair is gone.**

**Return to methods.**

*Figure 3.1* Screenshot A of Author 3's Twine Story.

### Hypertext Theory

Hypertext—or digital data interconnected by a reader's click or finger tap—has come to embody the very inherent structure of the internet. Astrid Ensslin argues in her chapter in *The Oxford Encyclopedia of Literary Theory* entitled "Hypertext Theory" that the linguistic roots of the term hypertext paint a picture for the term's meaning related to the rhizomatic connection of networks. The term hypertext is rooted in the Greek *hypér* translating to "over" or "beyond" and the Latin term *texere*, meaning "to weave" (Ensslin, "Hypertext Theory" 2). Ensslin explains that hypertext networks online utilize the connective protocol of the digital, which is Hypertext Markup Language (HTML). Where the traditional method of hypertext navigation was limited to a mouse click, newer approaches incorporate "mouse-over, touch, controller buttons, voice recognition, or even head position and vision direction (as in the case of VR)" (Ensslin "Hypertext Theory" 2). Hypertext creates diverging paths between text segments, often referred to as *nodes*, and later relabelled as *lexias*. As Ensslin argues, a typical hypertext lexia includes one or more hypertexts which allows readers to select various pathways with each reading, thereby creating distinct mental images of the text or even alternative textual manifestations. ("Hypertext Theory" 3). This interconnected data forms large masses of networked information online and it creates the very basic structures of digital tools we use every day including social media platforms, search engines and email.

The genesis of hypertext theory is typically identified as a moment in 1965 when information technology scholar Theodor Nelson coined the term *hypertext* in his lectures at Vassar College. He referred to hypertext as "non-sequential writing—text that branches and allows choices to the reader, best read at an interactive screen. As popularly conceived, this is a series of text chunks connected by links which offer the reader different pathways" (Ensslin "Hypertext Theory" 2). Nelson went on to argue that the capabilities of hypertext would stretch the margins of what was possible with information learning. He saw hypertext as a method that would define the future because it seemingly paralleled the branching ways in which humans form thought processes. Nelson argued that the boundless, interactive capability of hypertext would begin to infiltrate all structures of knowledge.

Laura Okkema argues in her work entitled "Hearing the Voices of the Deserters: Activist Critical Making in Electronic Literature" that Nelson envisioned hypertext becoming the very foundation of learning where the hierarchies and divisions of disciplines would dissolve because "all those who can read would be able to read everything" (Okkema 29). For Nelson, a move towards information as hypertext was urgent as he believed the way in which society approached information processing was incongruent with the inherent rhizomatic nature of knowledge—and, in this sense, our progress as a culture was diminishing. Nelson's belief in the possibilities of hypertext is immortalized in Robert Coover's 1992 article for *The New York Times* entitled "The End of Books." Coover outlines the potentiality of learning with hypertext and describes the championing of its supporters: "You will often hear them proclaim, quite seriously, that there have been three great events in the history of literacy: the invention of writing, the invention of movable type and the invention of hypertext" (Coover). Coover hones in on the ways in which the scholarly value of hypertext, at the time, began to shift by framing the medium as a significant form of literature. From here, hypertext was not only appreciated as a tool to engage with information learning but also a method for storytelling, particularly in a nonfiction sense.

Nelson's legacy of hypertext as a transformative, empowering structure went on to infiltrate belief systems around digital studies for decades. The field of hypertext literature has been categorized scholarly, similar to the feminist movement, in waves. Scholars in the first wave of digital humanities, such as George P. Landow and David J. Bolter, contributed to a sentiment that hypertext produces liberation because of its inherent capabilities. This sentiment was bolstered by Jane Yellowlees Douglas in her 1992 article "What Hypertexts Can Do That Print Narratives Cannot," which argues that hypertext shifts agency from the author to the reader of the text who now has the capability to choose the path of information. As Okkema claims, the scholarly sentiment around hypertext was that it inherently dissolved hierarchies of power through its democratic and at times anarchic disposition (29). These perspectives on hypertext were emerging alongside prominent scholarly affinities with poststructuralist and deconstructivist theoretical frameworks. As Ensslin and Skains suggest in their 2017 chapter "Hypertext: Storyspace to Twine" in *The Bloomsbury Handbook of Electronic Literature*, theories such as "anti-logo centrism, the writerly text, the death of the author, decentring and non-closure" all contributed to hypertext's image as a gatekeeper of reader empowerment (5).

The scholarly take-up of hypertext literature in the late 1980s to 1990s, which was working through academia's strong affinity with poststructuralism, was the very essence of the *lexia* as a rhizome realized, or as Ensslin argues, "ramifying, decentralized, horizontally organized root structures, which do not have a clear beginning or end. Rhizomes conveniently deviate from the arborescent, hierarchical structures associated with logocentrism" ("Hypertext Theory" 4). This sentiment of nonlinearity was paralleling academia's poststructuralist stride, where hypertext theories of this time sought to challenge textual hierarchies in favour of subversive, avant-garde, and individualized reading experiences (Ensslin, "Hypertext Theory" 4). Ultimately, hypertext was positioned as transcending a data information organizer to embody a tool for political change.

However, second-wave scholars of hypertext, emerging in the 2000s, have cautiously tempered the previous overenthusiastic views of the medium's capabilities. In fact, scholars such as Ensslin, Pope, Miall, Dobson, Mangen and van der Weel have illuminated hypertext's potentially counter-liberating structure. In the same way previous scholars highlighted the reader's agency in being able to choose where to "go" next, contemporary hypertext scholars note that the writer still creates boundaries of choice. The hypertext writer builds the structure of the text and is able to anticipate every possible reading path. As Ensslin and Skains note, hypertexts have been found to, at times, serve a delimiting rather than empowering function for readers, stemming from the ways in which the text may cause confusion, serendipity and cognitive overload for those not accustomed to hypertextual forms of creative writing (5).

It seems that previous claims of hypertext's liberatory potential were exaggerated. This liberatory potential is not lost, however, it merely requires careful methodological analysis. As Ensslin argues by noting that hypertext and other forms of electronic, digital-born writing necessitate distinct, medium-specific hermeneutic frameworks, they actually work to acknowledge that hypertexts are never read in the same way twice. Their inherently fluid and personalized meanings depend on multiple re-readings by the reader/player ("Hypertext Theory" 4). Scholars of the second wave of hypertext concluded that the emancipatory potential of hypertext is subtler than previously theorized, but nevertheless present and strengthened by writing that is informed by immersive, adaptable and user-friendly practices (Ensslin and Skains 8). This emancipatory potential becomes heightened through hypertexts that are able to adopt co-creation modalities where the reader becomes a participant in the text's creation (Enslin and Skains 5). In these cases, subject boundaries break down between *reader* and *writer* where authorship is a collaborative process.

In 2010, Alice Bell published *The Possible Worlds of Hypertext Fiction* which details one of the most prominent methodological frameworks for analyzing hypertext literature. Bell applies Marie-Laure Ryan's 1991 model for possible worlds theory, as articulated in Ryan's book *Possible Worlds, Artificial Intelligence and Narrative Theory*, to a selection of Storyspace—a literary hypertext software—hypertext literatures in order to explore ontological self-consciousness (Bell 7). Bell suggests that when analyzing fictional texts, we must be attuned to how fictional stories actually work to produce alternate ontological networks. Bell argues that an ontological perspective is particularly useful because it facilitates a systematic exploration of the relationship between the reader and the hypertext in the real world, alongside the interaction with fictional agents, including characters and narrators, within the fictional realm ("Ontological Boundaries" 69). Ryan's theory suggests that our lives in relation to fictional texts can be organized by the categories of our *actual world* versus our *textual universe* (Bell and Ryan, *Possible Worlds* viii).

These categorical spheres split further to incorporate alternate possible worlds where the character of the story (our self in the case of the actual world) projects their hopes, dreams and wishes. Bell argues that her approach to possible worlds theory is not attempting to decipher between events of textual description that are ontologically illogical or not, but rather, she is interested in understanding how ontological structures are textually constructed (*Possible Worlds* 26). Applying Bell's possible worlds theory to the *Click Me* research is complex because the model explored in her book is contingent on fictional worlds created through text. This poses the question of how nonfictional writing, such as hypertext illness narratives, might be analyzed by paying attention to ontological construction. Although Bell draws a line between fiction and nonfiction, there is more to explore in the seeming construction of "truth" found in nonfiction accounts, particularly when considering the ways in which telling one's story through experience can blur our understanding of informational reality.

In Hayles' "Print is Flat, Code is Deep: The importance of media-specific analysis," the author calls on scholars to conceptualize text as an embodied entity of materiality. This materiality is a dynamic attribute that arises from the interaction between the text as a physical object, its conceptual substance, and the interpretive processes of readers and writers (Hayles, "Print is Flat" 72). For Hayles, the materiality of hypertext is something that cannot be predetermined, but rather, is formed in its relationality to the reader. In later works, such as *My Mother was a Computer: Digital Subjects and Literary Texts*, Hayles sharpens her perspective on textual materiality as an emergent property constituted through the relationality between material characteristics and signifying strategies (3). In this sense, it becomes significant to distinguish between physicality and materiality, where the latter embodies the meaning-making processes produced through the former's relationality with signification. In other words, materiality is about meaning. When the reader engages with the text, the materiality of the relationship is born through interactivity. Hayles argues that the materiality of hypertext is not the physicality of the text, but rather, more akin to "connective tissue" that bridges together the physical and the interpretive or "the artifact and the user" ("Print is Flat" 72). Hayles digs into the ramifications of hypertext theory being born from the poststructuralist movement by calling into question the linguistic turn's framing of text as immaterial verbal construction. This ideology works to produce the Cartesian mind–body split by seemingly erasing the physicality of the text rather than viewing the material and the abstract as integrated.

This Cartesian framing has real implications, according to Hayles, as it works to separate class and economic factors with the project of creation.

This is how the politics of the production, publication and dissemination of texts can be separated from the textual creation of the author. As Hayles argues "We can no longer afford to pretend that texts are immaterial or that text on screen is the same as text in print. The immateriality of the text has ceased to be a useful or even a viable fiction" ("Print is Flat" 86–87). Hayles' work is foundational for working with the *Click Me* research because it highlights the complexities of the politics of text production. This is a topic explored in depth in later sections of this chapter devoted to the Twine Revolution in relation to the accessibility of electronic literature for marginalized identities. Hayles' work, ultimately, reinforces that the materiality of hypertext includes the meaning-making processes of interaction between the physical and the signification of language.

Finally, the third wave of hypertext scholarship, as described by Ensslin, actually precedes the second wave, yet has only recently been adopted more prolifically ("Hypertext Theory" 5). This third wave is turning more directly to the experiences of hypertext readers. This research is novel and ongoing, and it seeks to explore the multitude of ways readers process the rhizomatic, multimodal elements of digital-born literature. This scholarly turn to the experience of readers is promising, however, I wonder about ways to explore the experience of writers as well. Particularly, how are authors experiencing the act of creating hypertext fictions in relation to their illness? The state of the literature on hypertext resides at an interesting crossroads, almost anticipating research that will look deeper into what it means to be a hypertext author. Where the current scholarly focus on hypertext centres readers and the experience of reading, navigating and clicking hypertexts, this book intends to shift the discussion towards the experience of writing hypertexts. The scholarly field of illness narratives has taken an approach to understanding the embodied practice of writing about one's experience of illness and questioning how this might be therapeutic for the author. This same sentiment seems to be missing from the literature on hypertext.

## Electronic Literature

Literary hypertext, a genre of digital-born writing, is situated within a larger field known as electronic literature. Electronic literature is described by Scott Rettberg in his book *Electronic Literature* as new and emerging forms of writing and narrative that play with the relationality between the computer and the network in ways that contend that literature could not exist without the influence of digital culture (11). The genre has grown significantly from the 1990s to the present day as the capabilities of technology expand and grow. The term electronic literature has been contested in the field for decades, with scholars offering alternatives that they believe capture the essence of the described works more accurately. As Rettberg explains, scholar John Cayley put forward "writing in networked and programmable media" (11) whereas other scholars value narrower adherences such as *hypertext* (Nelson; Landow), *cybertext* (Aarseth), or *e-poetry* (Glazier). Nevertheless, electronic literature as a descriptor has prevailed, likely due to its generality and ability to represent newer modes of digital storytelling. Rettberg defines forms of electronic literature in expansive ways including hypertext fiction and poetry, digital art installations, and even narratives generated by artificial intelligence or conversational characters known as chatterbots (Rettberg 13). As we see, the first category encompasses the medium of this book. Yet, electronic literature can account for a robust collection of modalities and approaches to literary creation.

Today, the dominant understanding of electronic literature is refined to include the notion of, Hayles' term, *born-digital* creations. Electronic literature, at its core, is difficult to reproduce or distribute on the print page because its origins are within the dynamic space of the digital. Works of electronic literature tend to rely on code, digital interactivity or computer generation, to tell a story whereas the confines of print media are typically unable to produce the same results. But more significantly, at the root of electronic literature is a disruption of print conventions. Not only is electronic literature unable to be translated into print, but it also challenges the boundaries of the static medium. For instance, electronic literature's affinity with the term *reader/player* to describe the agent who engages with the text speaks to the genre's resistance to the boundaries of long-standing axioms where a text can be a game, a narrative, a work of art, etc. Where print media may rely on linearity, electronic literature turns to the malleability of the digital to explore multiplicity, interactivity and rhizomatic structures.

We see this in the electronic literature projects of UK-based artist Christine Wilks that utilize multimodality in the form of text and images to explore autobiographical undercurrents of pressurized normative femininity with harmful expectations of gender roles enforced through society and family. Wilks' Flash fiction *Underbelly* (2010) is influenced by the sociohistorical landscape of northern England. In her work, Wilks explores her sister's identity as a stone-carving artist through the setting of a former colliery's industrial past. Auditory and textual elements of 19th-century female coal miners weave together with a storyline of a contemporary woman sculptor. As the reader/player, you soon plunge into the world of *Underbelly*, an underworld of female-gendered anatomy where you may shift through a uterus canal or play a Wheel of Fortune-style game of pregnancy fate. A textual element bombards you to "Choose! Choose!" as "Time is running out." You may play the game multiple times and never receive the same outcome. But in all versions, the story urges the reader/player to confront internalized perceptions of gender roles, compulsory motherhood and fertility.

The future of electronic literature is expansive. As this project argues, there are dynamic and novel capabilities for one of the more traditional subgenres of electronic literature, literary hypertext, especially when looking at therapeutic, digital illness narratives. However, other more innovative adaptations of electronic literature are moving away from storytelling through a computer screen or a smartphone to the VR visor. VR technology is in its infancy, however recently, more accessible, wearable VR technology, such as the Oculus Quest (Meta Platforms), is opening up the medium, in some ways, for the common consumer. Among VR video games, social connection spaces, virtual movie screenings and virtual workspaces is a budding medium of VR electronic literature.

*Down the Rabbit Hole*, for example, is a 2019 VR game developed by Cortopia Studios. As the reader/player, you navigate immersive tableaus, familiar to the world of Lewis Carroll's 1865 *Alice's Adventures in Wonderland*, that wrap around your body through VR graphics. You play as a young girl who is in search of her lost pet. Where *Down the Rabbit Hole* differs from some VR video games is through its textual and story-based choose-your-own-adventure plot. As you solve various riddles and puzzles to gain access to the next setting, the narrator of the story will show you a selection of cards imprinted with choices. The narrator may ask your name, what type of animal your lost pet is, or how you should interact with certain characters. Selecting a card drives the story in diverging directions which gives the reader/player differing outcomes. The experience *Down the Rabbit Hole* reinforces most drastically is electronic literature's disruption of the conventions of print media and the genre's embracing of new technological developments. Ultimately, electronic literature is an expansive and growing field that encompasses a multitude of forms.

## Literary Hypertext and Rhizomatic Multiplicity

In the 1990s, as hypertext technologies began to grow, so too did the practice of literary hypertext and games that utilize hypertext features. In 1993, Macintosh released one of the most successful computer games of the time, *Myst*. The puzzle adventure game was written using Hypercard, a hypermedia system that predates the emergence of the World Wide Web. *Myst* was built using the intricate layering of a series of Hypercard stacks and became one of the most popular interactive fiction games of the time. It now has been reimagined in VR as a newly released Oculus Quest game. Near the end of the millennium, literary hypertext technology was becoming increasingly accessible to game developers, scholars and individuals as a media artefact to study and create with. Today, there is a plethora of literary hypertext software available to everyday users, most notably Twine—the tool utilized by the *Click Me* authors which will be discussed in depth below.

Digital hypertext responds, ultimately, to a disillusionment with static, linear digital writing, such as online articles and e-books. As hypertext scholars McAdams and Berger argue, an innovative process for both reading and writing is required for narratives born in the online space to match the notion of multiplicity inherent in the digital medium. Dominant conceptualizations of literary hypertext, however, tend to make structural assumptions that the medium exclusively represents rhizomatic, fictional narratives. For example, McAdams and Berger suggest that when the structure of online writing becomes a fixed copy of that which can be produced on a piece of paper, we lose the digital capability of agency in navigation. The reader, then, has no choice but to follow the path of the narrative as it has been revealed to them. In contrast, the authors argue that hypertext literature can embody a myriad of narrative paths for the reader/player to explore. These assumptions of narrative multiplicity, however, fail to represent all forms of literary hypertext as many do, in fact, follow a linear path.

Most scholarly contributions on literary hypertext have been concentrated in the realm of fiction. Classified as forms of digital fiction, hypertexts can tell a story in ways that play with the reader's sense of intervention. Hypertextual forms of digital fiction tend to exhibit characteristics of games, and for this reason, have been taken up thoroughly in scholarly game studies. Stemming from its accessibility in creation and counterhegemonic form, hypertext digital fictions have been both taken up and pioneered by subjugated communities to share stories that are typically veered to the margins. For example, the critically significant digital fiction *Queers in Love at the End of the World* by Anna Anthropy tells a ten-second story of a world being catapulted into emptiness. As the reader/player, you are up against a clock with a series of hypertext choices describing how you wish to interact with your lover before the whole world is "wiped away." *Queers in Love* uses multilinear narrativity in ways that foreground tenderness and compassion against a backdrop of impending destruction. Similarly, *Known Unknowns* is a hypertext digital fiction that tells the story of Nadia Nazari, a high school student dealing with the motivations of her ex-best friend, hunting for ghost raccoons, and contemplating Queer desire. Found at the core of both fictions is the desire to give narrative voice to a subjugated identity through reflexive interaction between the story and the reader.

As noted above, much of the scholarly work on literary hypertext is focused on the medium as rhizomatic, fictional narrative. As Ensslin argues in *Canonizing Hypertext*:

> Essentially, the abstract idea of 'hyper-text' is based on the rhizome metaphor (Deleuze and Guattari, 1987), characterized by a ramifying, horizontally organized root structure, which is, unlike arborescent structures, decentralized, i.e. there is no core, or 'trunk', and no visible hierarchy. (11)

It is significant for the *Click Me* research to first question what we mean when we label a narrative as rhizomatic. Mainly, does this assume different plot options that can be realized through the choices of the reader, or are there novel ways we can interpret multiplicity in a relatively "linear" hypertext narrative? As will be discussed in depth in Chapter 4, the Twine illness narratives that the *Click Me* authors designed embodied the rhizome in different ways. Every story, though, has a single opening passage. Many narratives had a hierarchical, linear structure, as well. Despite this, there is something about the concept of the rhizome in connection to hypertext that allows for a deeper consideration of different kinds of ways to read multiplicity in the narratives.

I consider the potential of literary hypertext as a tool to write stories of nonfiction—particularly illness narratives. McAdams and Berger argue that innovative digital writing practices are not just desirable but essential for advancing journalistic, nonfiction and even scholarly writing in ways enabled by hypertext. The authors suggest that hypertext should be more comprehensively adopted in nonfiction communities because it improves the reading experience of those engaging with the work. McAdams and Berger argue that unilinear storytelling becomes saturated in value judgments. Here, the author becomes the gatekeeper of meaning by choosing the structure of ideas and in "a well-crafted hypertext, readers immediately select what matters most to them" (McAdams and Berger). Meaning can be coded in multiple ways but includes the order of ideas, the amount of text devoted to a topic, or the author's decisions about which ideas to omit. Further, meaning is cultivated through a normative story structure that steers a course through a beginning, middle and end. In the limitless story space of literary hypertext, there can be multiple paths to both enter and exit the story with a rhizomatic internal structure. However, it becomes evident that the structure of hypertext literature does not resist every limitation of linear writing, as described by McAdams and Berger. Even with hypertext choice for the reader, literary hypertext is still confined to the structure and boundaries created by the author of the text.

Some hypertext scholars, such as Astrid Ensslin and Alice Bell, have noted that reading literary hypertext in isolation does not produce empowerment or freedom for the reader in itself. In fact, the consumption of literary hypertext removed from the creation process may render notions of restriction (Ensslin, *Canonizing Hypertext* 3). It is through the process of collaborative reading, discussion and creation of literary hypertext, Ensslin argues, where empowerment in narrative multiplicity is born (*Canonizing Hypertext* 3). It seems that when we break down normative, hegemonic practices of writing for the purpose of empowerment, we must also consider deconstructing the binary of *reader* and *writer*. Perhaps it is when the identity of *reader* becomes amalgamated with that of *creator* that the restrictive structure of linear narrativity breaks down. From a place situating literary hypertext as a subversion to normative ways of both reading and writing, this book considers where illness narratives can be taken up in the medium. It will be significant for this project to explore why literary hypertext might be beneficial, particularly for women and nonbinary people with hyperandrogenism. Perhaps, when being coded as an "abnormally" sexed body in our world becomes an act of subverting binaries of biological sex, responses that aim to empower these individuals must match this undermining of institutional and societal norms. These norms may include our standard practices of writing and reading illness narratives.

## Twinery.org

Twine is one software for literary hypertext design. There is a legacy of hypertext systems, though, that has preceded the development of Twine and other current tools for building hypertext stories. These programs tend to adopt a similar scheme called a *directed path*, reminiscent of a rhizome of boxes and lines, which a reader is intended to move through from one textual unit, a *node*, to another (Moulthrop and Salter 51). The term *node* has evolved through various eras of hypertext itself, being replaced by the term *lexia* by hypertext pioneer George P. Landow, and later various labels such as tweet or post (Moulthrop and Salter 51). Twine names the *node* as a *passage*, and this is the language this book will use to refer to a textual unit of literary hypertext. To further complicate things, the passage as a textual unit may not always include text. A passage can house an image, video or sound cues and a reader can be brought to the next passage via a programmed timer. This, however, is not the typical way passages are designed. Twine's collectively designed instructional guide, the Twine Cookbook, refers to passages as "divisions of time, space, or combinations of the two. They can also be thought of as blocks of dialogue, sections of code, or simply ways to break up a complicated project into more easily understood parts." Most likely, a passage will include text and at least one hypertext link. A *link* is the final critical term that builds the foundation of a hypertext story.

According to Moulthrop and Salter, the always-online nature of our lives has led us to become familiar with links as a word, or a phrase, distinguished by a unique colour and typically underlined, that signals the user to click or tap it. These visual traces, according to the authors, are only the top layer of a deeply complex process. A link may refer to a number of parts including the anchoring text, the housed string of code, the structural image of the connecting line in the Twine's interface, or an action. The final definition, according to Moulthrop and Salter, is the most significant for understanding literary hypertext (53). A link triggers an action that makes a change. In the context of a Twine story, typically a link will transition the reader to a new passage. This book will refer to Twine's links as *hypertext, hyperlink* or *hypertext link* depending on the context. For example, *hypertext* is used when referring to text in a passage that houses a link, *hyperlink* refers to the link housed within the text or the action of linking as a verb, in the case of *hyperlinked. Hypertext link* is used in an attempt to refer to the text, link and action together.

In the past two decades, Twine has cultivated a movement of support from marginalized game developers who are often excluded from masculinist, white spaces of game development (Anthropy 90; Harvey 96). Twine is a culture of free production and distribution. The tool is free to download, open-source and can export stories as HTML files to be published online. It is also regarded as user-friendly as no coding knowledge is required by the author to build a basic hypertext story. Beyond technological and financial accessibility, literary hypertexts created in Twine have the potential to subvert assumed norms in traditional narrative mediums by promoting experimentation through multiple endings, branching plots and interactive components (Harvey 101).

Developed by interactive fiction author Chris Klimas in 2009 to reduce barriers to entry for storytellers of marginalized identities, Twine hypertext technology was selected for the *Click Me* research because the storytelling engine is free with an internet connection. But beyond that, the interface and process to write a basic hypertext story is relatively intuitive. Instructions found in the opening passage of the interface advise the user to enclose text within double square brackets to create a hypertext to another passage. Although, critically, moving beyond the basics swiftly becomes inaccessible for the inexperienced and this is a barrier to entry for hypertext creation as a whole. For illness narratives, branching hypertext has the potential as a productive platform for authors to learn how power functions in their stories[4] as they build in narrative choices that yield consequences (Greco 85). Literary hypertext has been taken up in game studies as a platform that blows open access to game design for marginalized communities, and I began to wonder how this promise of access could translate for women and nonbinary people with hyperandrogenism to write and publish illness narratives.

Twine has become a home for subjugated, Queered, racialized or gendered identities to occupy space in gaming and digital literary communities (Bernardi; Friedhoff). The platform has come to be described by scholars as a predominately "queer- and women-dominated" community that has facilitated the "democratization of hypertext" as a narrative form (Ensslin and Skains 10). The literary texts created using Twine are typically fiction or digital games, however, a smaller subset of Twines feature nonfiction narrative.

For example, *Find the Woman of Colour at the Indie Game Jam* is a Twine narrative by Sui Sea "based on a true story" and "tagged" by the author as a nonfiction piece. As the reader, you follow along with the author's experience as a sole Woman of Colour at a "game jam" populated by men and white women who continually reassert the author's identity as Other. In the story, you encounter the following scene: "you step into the hackerspace and cringe. nearly everyone is a dude, and 99% of them are white. you blink. where are the women?" The latter question is marked as hypertext that leads you further into the narrative. *Find the Woman of Colour* demonstrates how Twine is used to write nonfiction stories about the experience of marginalization—a sentiment critical to this project.

## Game Creators at the Margins: #GamerGate and the Twine Revolution

The issues of sexism and exclusion have been at the heart of public game creation for decades, particularly in literary hypertext games. Because this book claims literary hypertext as a space of accessibility for marginalized individuals to tell their stories, it is vital to devote space, here, to large-scale movements of exclusion in the game-creation community, particularly in relation to hypertext. Sarah Einstein and Matthew Vetter discuss in their article "Women Writing in Digital Spaces: Engaging #Gamergate and Twine in the Gender Studies-Composition Course" the details surrounding a social media controversy and campaign known as #GamerGate. Einstein and Vetter argue "At the heart of this attack was a construction of 'gamer' as an essentialized identity; one that is male, socially conservative, and anti-feminist." In August of 2014, a sexist campaign of harassment began to proliferate in the online gaming community that targeted specifically female game developers Zoë Quinn and Brianna Wu, as well as feminist journalist Anita Sarkeesian. The campaign was initiated by Quinn's ex-partner, Eron Gjoni, who penned a defaming blog post that accused Quinn of engaging in an unethical relationship with a gaming journalist named Nathan Grayson. Gjoni falsely argued that the massive success of Quinn's popular hypertext story-game, *Depression Quest*, was due to her taking advantage of a relationship with a journalist to cultivate a series of praising commentaries on her project. Proponents of #GamerGate also criticized Quinn's fundraising of *Depression Quest* via the platform Patreon.

Massive support of Gjoni's blog post has been described as a right-wing backlash to increasing progressiveness or "wokeness" in the gaming community (O'Donnell 654; Dowling et al. 982; Mortensen and Sihvonen 1353). The response from Gjoni's supporters included doxing (publishing private or identifying information about an individual), threats of rape, and death threats against Quinn and other female game developers. Einstein and Vetter explore in their article ways to navigate the reality of sexism and exclusion in digital creation. They argue that women writing online encounter much more—and distinctly unique forms of—harassment than men, and the development of this new mediation of gendered violence is central to understanding why women do or do not participate in digital conversations and engagement (Einstein and Vetter). Writing this book in the shadow of #GamerGate leads me to recognize not only the kind of oppression women and nonbinary folks experience in the normative medical system but also the kind of harassment and gatekeeping they experience when they attempt to tell their stories in the digital space.

The #GamerGate movement unfolded several years after prolific literary hypertext creator Anna Anthropy wrote her 2012 book *Rise of the Videogame Zinesters: How Freaks, Normals, Amateurs, Artists, Dreamers, Drop-outs, Queers, Housewives, and People Like You Are Taking Back an Art Form*. Anthropy's book is the compass of the *Click Me* research. *Rise of the Videogame Zinesters* was one of the initial publications that identified a political movement in the DIY gaming industry spearheaded by marginalized writers. Her instructional manifesto became massively popular in the indie game creation community where identities who were typically silenced felt empowered by her call to action. In her book, Anthropy calls for the marginalized to organize and insert themselves into the gaming industry in ways that challenge traditionally normative methods of creation and dissemination of games. Specifically, she encourages the use of Twine. Anthropy summons her readers:

> There's nothing to stop us from making our voices heard now. And there will be plenty of voices. Among those voices heard, there will be plenty of mediocrity, and plenty of games that have no meaning to anyone outside the author and maybe her friends. We'll find new ways to sort that shit. And imagine what we'll gain; real diversity, a plethora of voices and experiences, and a new avenue for human beings to tell their stories and connect with other human beings. Are you excited?
>
> (161)

Anthropy saw hope in the accessibility and DIY nature of literary hypertext technology for all to share their stories. Ultimately, she became a proponent of the "Twine Revolution" or the democratization of game design by using the affordances of the Twine software. Ultimately, the promise and excitement in democratizing hypertext tools like Twine must also acknowledge that hypertext writing and publishing are relational and affective, with ripple effects that spread in secret and out loud, across multiple lives, and in ways that are difficult to trace.

## Notes

1 A breakdown of participant make-up, including identity markers, is outlined in Chapter 4.
2 A brief overview of the methodology used in the analysis of the data of this book is outlined in Chapter 4.
3 I am aware of my habitual use of the word "like," as shown by its instance nine times in the two presented quotes. However, I am retaining it here as a form of feminist protest.
4 The pedagogy aimed at narrative power and consequences is outlined in Chapter 4. Here, authors learned how power functions through the experience of hyperandrogenism as well as design principles of hypertext interactivity and multiple narrative paths, for example.

## Works Cited


Anthropy, Anna. *Rise of the Videogame Zinesters: How Freaks, Normals, Amateurs, Artists, Dreamers, Dropouts, Queers, Housewives, and People Like You Are Taking Back an Art Form*, 1st ed. Seven Stories Press, 2012.

Anthropy, Anna. *Queers in Love at the End of the World*. itch.io, 12 March 2016, https://w.itch.io/end-of-the-world

Aarseth, Espen J. *Cybertext: Perspectives on Ergodic Literature*. JHU Press, 1997.

Balsamo, Anne Marie. *Technologies of the Gendered Body: Reading Cyborg Women*. Duke University Press, 1996.

Barad, Karen. *Meeting the Universe Halfway: Quantum Physics and the Entanglement of Matter and Meaning*. Duke University Press, 2007.

Barad, Karen. "Ontological Boundaries and Methodological Leaps: The Importance of Possible Worlds Theory for Hypertext Fiction (and Beyond)." *New Narratives: Stories and Storytelling in the Digital Age*, edited by Ruth Page and Bronwen Thomas, UNP – Nebraska Paperback, 2011, pp. 63–82.

Barad, Karen. *The Possible Worlds of Hypertext Fiction*. Palgrave Macmillan, 2010.

Barad, Karen, and Marie-Laure Ryan. *Possible Worlds Theory and Contemporary Narratology*. University of Nebraska Press, 2019.

Bernardi, Joe. "Choose Your Own Adventure-Maker: Twine and the Art of Personal Games." *Motherboard*, 2013, http://motherboard.vice.com/blog/twine-and-the-art-of-personal-games

Bolter, David Jay. *Writing Space. Computers, Hypertext, and the Remediation of Print*. Routledge, 2001.

Braidotti, Rosi. "Four Theses on Posthuman Feminism." *Anthropocene Feminism*, edited by Richard Grusin, University of Minnesota Press, 2017, pp. 21–48.

Clough, Patricia T. "The Affective Turn: Political Economy, Biomedia and Bodies." *Theory, Culture & Society*, vol. 25, no. 1, 2008, pp. 1–22.

Coleman, Rebecca, et al. "Feminist New Materialist Practice: The Mattering of Methods." Special Issue of *MAI: Feminism & Visual Culture*, Summer, no. 4, 2019.

Coover, Robert. "The End of Books." *The New York Times*, 21 June 1992. http://www.nytimes.com/books/98/09/27/specials/coover-end.html

Cortopia Studios. *Down the Rabbit Hole*. Beyond Frames Entertainment, 26 March 2020, https://downtherabbitholegame.com/

Crenshaw, Kimberlé. "Demarginalizing the Intersection of Race and Sex: A Black Feminist Critique of Antidiscrimination Doctrine, Feminist Theory, and Antiracist Politics." *Feminist Legal Theory*, Routledge, 2018, pp. 57–80.

Cyan Worlds Inc. *Myst*. Cyan Worlds Inc, 26 August 2021.

Deleuze, Gilles, and Félix Guattari. *A Thousand Plateaus: Capitalism and Schizophrenia*. University of Minnesota Press, 1987.

Dolphijn, Rick, and Iris van der Tuin. *New Materialism: Interviews & Cartographies*, 1st ed. Open Humanities Press, 2012.

Douglas, Jane Yellowlees. "What Hypertexts Can Do That Print Narratives Cannot." *Reader: Essays in Reader-oriented Theory, Criticism, and Pedagogy*, vol. 28, 1992, pp. 1–22.

Dowling, David O., et al. "One Year of# GamerGate: The Shared Twitter Link as Emblem of Masculinist Gamer Identity." *Games and Culture*, vol. 15, no. 8, 2020, pp. 982–1003.

Einstein, Sarah and Matthew Vetter. "Women Writing in Digital Spaces: Engaging #Gamergate and Twine in the Gender Studies-Composition Course." *Digital Rhetoric Collaborative*, 7 May 2015, https://www.digitalrhetoriccollaborative.org/2015/05/07/women-writing-in-digital-spaces-engaging-gamergate-and-twine-in-the-gender-studies-composition-course/. Accessed 1 March 2021.

Ensslin, Astrid. *Canonizing Hypertext: Explorations and Constructions*. Continuum, 2007.

Ensslin, Astrid, and Lyle Skains. "Hypertext: Storyspace to Twine." *The Bloomsbury Handbook of Electronic Literature*, edited by Joseph Tabbi, Bloomsbury Publishing, 2017, pp. 295–310.

Ensslin, Astrid. "Hypertext Theory." *The Oxford Encyclopedia of Literary Theory*, edited by John Frow, et al., Oxford University Press, 2020.

Friedhoff, Jane. "Untangling Twine: A Platform Study." In: *Proceedings of DiGRA 2013: DeFragging Game Studies*, Atlanta, GA. http://www.digra.org/wp-content/uploads/digital-library/paper_67.compressed.pdf

Glazier, Loss Pequeño. *Digital Poetics: The Making of E-Poetries*. University of Alabama Press, 2001.

Greco, Diane. "Hypertext with Consequences: Recovering a Politics of Hypertext." *Association for Computing Machinery*, 1996, pp. 85–92

Haraway, Donna J. "A Cyborg Manifesto: Science, Technology, and Socialist-Feminism in the Late Twentieth Century." *Simians, Cyborgs, and Women: The Reinvention of Nature*, Routledge, 1991, pp. 149–181.

Haraway, Donna J. "Playing String Figures with Companion Species." Donna J. Haraway (Ed.), *Staying with the Trouble. Making Kin in the Chthulucene*, Duke University Press, 2016, pp. 9–29.

Harvey, Allison. "Twine's Depoliticization, and the Queering of Design." *Game*, no. 3, 2014.

Hayles, N. Katherine. *My Mother Was a Computer: Digital Subjects and Literary Texts*. University of Chicago Press, 2005.

Hayles, N. Katherine. "Print is Flat, Code is Deep: The Importance of Media-Specific Analysis." *Poetics Today*, vol. 25, no. 1, 2004, pp. 67–90.

Hennessy, Brendan Patrick. *Known Unknowns*. Izzy Marbella (Art), 2016, https://known.zone/credits

Hird, Myra J. *Sex, Gender, and Science*. Palgrave Macmillan, 2004.

Klimas, Chris. *Twine*. The Interactive Technology Foundation, 2009, http://twinery.org/

Landow, George P. *Hypertext 3.0*. John Hopkins University Press, 2006.

Mangen, Anne and Adriaan van der Weel. "Why Don't We Read Hypertext Novels?" *Convergence*, vol. 23, no. 2, 2017, pp. 166–181.

McAdams, Mindy and Stephanie Berger. "Hypertext." *The Journal of Electronic Publishing*, vol. 6, no. 3, 2001. Online Journal.

Miall, David and Teresa Dobson. "Reading Hypertext and the Experience of Literature." *Journal of Digital Information*, vol. 2, no. 1, 2001. Online Journal.

Mortensen, Torill Elvira, and Tanja Sihvonen. "Negative Emotions Set in Motion: The Continued Relevance of #GamerGate." *The Palgrave Handbook of International Cybercrime and Cyberdeviance*, edited by Thomas J. Holt and Adam M. Bossler, Palgrave Macmillan, 2020, pp.1353–1374.

Moulthrop, Stuart. *Victory Garden*. Eastgate Systems, 1992.

Nelson, Theodor H. *Literary Machines: The Report on, and of, Project Xanadu Concerning Word Processing, Electronic Publishing, Hypertext, Thinkertoys, Tomorrow's Intellectual Revolution, and Certain Other Topics Including Knowledge, Education and Freedom*. Mindful Press, 1993.

O'Donnell, Jessica. "Militant Meninism: The Militaristic Discourse of Gamergate and Men's Rights Activism." *Media, Culture & Society*, vol. 42, no. 5, 2020, pp. 654–674.

Okkema, Laura. *Hearing the Voices of the Deserters: Activist Critical Making in Electronic Literature*. University of Central Florida, PhD dissertation, 2019.

Pitts-Taylor, Victoria. *The Brain's Body: Neuroscience and Corporeal Politics*. Duke University Press, 2016.

Plant, Sadie. "On the Matrix: Cyberfeminist Simulations." *The Gendered Cyborg: A Reader*, edited by Hovenden, Fiona, et al., Routledge, 2000, pp. 265–275.

Pope, James. "A Future for Hypertext Fiction." *Convergence*, vol. 12, no. 4, 2006, pp. 447–465.

Puar, Jasbir K. "'I Would Rather Be a Cyborg Than a Goddess': Becoming-Intersectional in Assemblage Theory." *philoSOPHIA: A Journal of Continental Feminism*, vol. 2, no. 1, 2012, pp. 49–66.

Quinn, Zoë. *Depression Quest*. The Quinnspiracy, 14 February 2013, http://www.depressionquest.com/

Rettberg, Scott. *Electronic Literature*. Polity Press, 2019.

Richardson, Rick T., et al. "Color and Contrast in E-Learning Design: A Review of the Literature and Recommendations for Instructional Designers and Web Developers." *MERLOT Journal of Online Learning and Teaching*, vol. 10, no. 4, 2014, pp. 657–670.

Ryan, Marie-Laure. *Possible Worlds, Artificial Intelligence, and Narrative Theory*. Indiana University Press, 1991.

Salter, Anastasia, and Stuart Moulthrop. *Twining*. Amherst College Press, 2021.

Sanzo, Kameron. "New Materialism(s)." *Critical Posthumanism*, 25 April 2018, https://criticalposthumanism.net/new-materialisms/. Accessed 19 February 2020.

Sea, Sui. *Find the Woman of Colour at the Indie Game Jam*. Itch.io, 9 January 2016, https://sui.itch.io/woc. Accessed 5 December 2022.

Smith, Daniel and John Protevi. "Gilles Deleuze." *The Stanford Encyclopedia of Philosophy* (Spring 2020 Edition), edited by Edward N. Zalta, 23 May 2008, https://plato.stanford.edu/archives/spr2020/entries/deleuze/. Accessed 22 February 2021.

Truman, Sarah E. "Feminist New Materialisms." *SAGE Research Methods*, 2020.

*Twine Cookbook*. Twinery.org, 2021, https://twinery.org/cookbook/

Wilks, Christine. *Underbelly*. Interactive Game, 2010, https://crissxross.net/elit/underbelly

# 4 How to DIY a Hypertext Illness Narrative Module

## Getting Started

If you only read one chapter of this book, I hope you choose this one, if only to speak to the affective nature of this project and the hope that it can incite the writing of more illness narratives. In this chapter I outline a framework for designing a hypertext illness narrative module using Twine. The *Click Me* module detailed here is intended to stand as a pedagogical tool for clinicians and researchers to build their own narrative therapy-based modules for patients in need (envisioned as individuals with hyperandrogenism, but there is also significant potential in the applications of hypertext therapy for other pathologized identities). That being said, individuals with hyperandrogenism or other nuances of biological sex embodiments who are seeking new ways, beyond the normative healthcare system, to respond to their illness can also find value in this guide. If you belong to this group, you may choose to focus on Figure 4.2 and start your reading from there. This figure presents the writing prompt offered to authors during the free writing portion of the *Click Me* illness narrative module, which may offer you inspiration to build your own story. Better yet, you can complete the *Click Me* module yourself by accessing it on itch.io, a platform for hosting indie games and other forms of electronic literature. You can access the module directly in your browser at this link: https://mperram.itch.io/twine-writing-module.

Writing a static print guide for a digital tool poses some notable challenges mainly that links break, digital tools evolve and software updates. *Click Me* authors used the 2.3.8 release of Twine in the Harlowe 3.1.0 story format (more to come on story formats later in this chapter, but generally Twine currently has four story format options, with one proofing format, and each holds a distinct visual layout, set of macros and internal JavaScript functionality). At the time this book was published, the latest version of Twine was 2.10.0, which utilizes Harlowe 3.3.9 as the default story format,

DOI: 10.4324/9781003646921-4

and was released on November 24, 2024. While the foundational principles discussed in this chapter will remain applicable, it is important to identify that certain technical aspects have evolved in the latest release. The Twine module framework presented in this chapter intentionally sidesteps tethering the instructions to any specific technical programming elements of Twine, or a specific story format, for that matter. My intention for this chapter is to outline a framework that prioritizes the development of content, framing, pedagogy and narrative exercises for a Twine module, as a way to uphold a sentiment of adaptability so that this guide may remain useful beyond Twine.

Twine, as discussed in length in Chapter 3, is designed with accessibility at the forefront. Authors can build basic narratives, even branching narratives, without the need for incorporating any substantive coding elements. Authors do have the option to enrich their narrative with more advanced programming elements such as variables, conditional logic, images, CSS and JavaScript. If you have the background, or perhaps the wherewithal to learn these programming advancements, there is a world of resources to support your designs. If this sounds like you, you may want to become familiar with the (https://twinery.org/cookbook/index.html), which offers a guide on choosing a story format and provides solutions for accomplishing common tasks with each of Twine's built-in formats. But, while on my accessibility soapbox, I want to invite those with little to no experience to the front of the crowd. This chapter is for you.

As a precursor to the content to come in this chapter, you really only need the following steps to make a Twine illness narrative module come to life—with the caveat that these steps align with the Twine 2.10.0 version:

1 Access Twinery.org

   a Open your web browser and navigate to https://twinery.org/.
   b Click on the "Use in your browser" button to access Twine directly in your browser. Alternatively, you can download the desktop application and install it to your device.

2 Create a New Story (an Individual Twine Project)

   a Once Twine is open, you will see a dashboard with options.
   b Select the "+New" button to create a new story.
   c A dialog box will appear prompting you to name your story. You can create a story that is named whatever you like (e.g., "My Hyperandrogenism Story").
   d Select "✓Create."

3 Create the First Passage

  a The story map view will appear where you can see and edit your story's structure.
  b You will see a default "Untitled Passage" in the centre of the screen. Double-click it to open.
  c You can rename the passage to something meaningful (e.g., "Start of my Hyperandrogenism Story") by clicking the "Rename" option in the top ribbon of the passage.
  d In the text area below, write the beginning of your story. For example: "Sixty-three. That's the number of hairs that [[shed]] from my scalp today."
  e The text enclosed in [[double square brackets]] creates links to new passages. In the example I provided, the new passage would be named "shed."

4 Build Your Story

  a Click the "X" in the top-right corner of the passage to go back to the story map view.
  b You will now see a new passage automatically created and linked based on the link you defined (i.e., "shed").
  c Now, you can double-click the new passage to edit its content and build out the narrative content of your story.

5 Save Your Story

  a If you are using the browser version of Twine, your stories are saved in your browser's local storage. This allows you to close the browser and return later to find your stories still available.
  b To create a backup, select "Build" in the top ribbon of the story map. Then select the "Publish to File" button which will save a copy of your story to your computer. This will download a .html file which you can upload later to continue editing.

6 Share Your Story

  a You can upload the .html file to any web hosting service to share your story online. The *Click Me* module I created is shared through itch.io.

To add more value to these basic steps, you may find it useful to refer to the Twine Reference (https://twinery.org/reference/en/). This guide offers detailed descriptions of Twine's user interface and introduces the broader "ecosystem" that it lives within. The Twine Reference touches on the vast landscape of possibilities that Twine promises, including basics of building a branching story to more complex features such as adding variables, using conditional logic, and incorporating multimedia elements—all of which I found useful in the development of my own illness narrative module.

## Designing the *Click Me* Research

There were four main stages to the research process of the study outlined in this book which include the *Click Me* module design phase, participant recruitment phase, experiment phase and data analysis phase. In the module design phase, I spent several months working with narrative therapy perspectives to develop a Twine module for writing literary hypertext illness narratives, of which the theoretical and technical aspects will be described in this chapter. The structure and efficacy of the module were the central objectives of the research design because the resource ultimately had to stand on its own as a pedagogical tool. The experiment phase of the research began at the start of the COVID-19 pandemic which saw social distancing mandates in effect. It was unsafe to be physically near the *Click Me* authors at this time, compounded by the fact that the authors were located expansively across Canada and beyond. The *Click Me* module had to facilitate the learning process in its entirety. Participants, of course, were directed to connect with me if they had questions, but it was important to mitigate any clarity issues at that base level so authors felt confident completing their stories on their own.

Participant recruitment for this study was completed over the course of a year through general calls for participants on public listservs, PCOS Facebook Groups, and PCOS subreddits (a centralized online group on the website Reddit, an online topic-based discussion community). The first line of contact with the *Click Me* authors was a recruitment poster posted in an online space. The poster depicts a pixelated image of an arcade game, to speak to Twine's affinity with game creation, with a neon title that reads: "Living with PCOS can be hard, especially when some symptoms challenge our ideas of what a feminine body should look like. Do you have a PCOS story to share? Writing about your experience can be empowering." The decision to centre the condition PCOS in the recruitment poster, and other onboarding documents, was intentional.

Receiving a formal diagnosis of hyperandrogenism is complex. Typically, patients will experience varying symptoms of hyperandrogenism, and upon medical investigation, are diagnosed with one of the many hyperandrogenism-related disorders (e.g., PCOS, Congenital Adrenal Hyperplasia, and Cushing's syndrome). It is not typical that patients are diagnosed with hyperandrogenism, in isolation, but rather if there are symptoms to suggest hyperandrogenism further diagnostic tests may be administered to identify an underlying disease (Oakley). Therefore, hyperandrogenism may not be a word that individuals are familiar with. PCOS, however, is the most common endocrine disorder among women of reproductive age (McGowan 289).

A significant number of individuals who experience PCOS experience symptoms of hyperandrogenism as well (Oakley). Therefore, in order to connect with a meaningful number of relevant participants, the recruitment for the study employed the language of PCOS instead of hyperandrogenism, where the latter was introduced and defined for participants later on.

It was critical for the *Click Me* study to take on this more complicated approach, rather than focusing on PCOS as a whole, for example, because the *Click Me* research is concerned with the experience of androgen excess and how that impacts one's relationship with gender presentation and cultural expectations. Using the disorder of PCOS alone, without the presence of hyperandrogenism, posed a problem because PCOS can produce a multitude of symptoms. For example, in this scenario, a participant with PCOS without hyperandrogenism could have experience with insulin resistance, obesity and, interestingly, skin tags. While these are important symptoms, they might not explicitly connect to the study's central themes around deviant femininity. The recruitment poster outlines three eligibility requirements, including that participants must be 18 years old or over, have the ability to speak and write in English, and have experienced elevated testosterone.

The *Click Me* study did not require a formal diagnosis of a disorder, or even elevated testosterone, from a physician. Interested participants who self-identify as having hyperandrogenism as per their lived experience with two or more symptoms were eligible (a list of symptoms will be detailed below). This distinction is critical because it opens up space for participation from individuals who may feel their concerns regarding symptoms have not been appropriately recognized within the patient–physician encounter. There was no maximum age range for this study as hyperandrogenism is a condition that affects individuals across their lifetimes and is found in many people transitioning into menopause. However, all the participants who completed the study were relatively young (between 21 and 36 years of age). This may be due to the digital recruitment method, the digital aspect of the study, or perhaps the age range that individuals are seeking to cope with their illness. This outcome requires further investigation.

I knew that, as a central part of this research, I wanted to look at the experiences of pathologized, "deviant" femininity. As detailed above, I needed participants who were struggling, either consciously or unconsciously, with the Queering of normative femininity. PCOS has an array of symptoms, and many people who have the disease have differing experiences. I knew I needed participants who were experiencing the symptoms of hyperandrogenism specifically (symptoms of excess testosterone). However, as discussed above, the issue with recruiting individuals with hyperandrogenism is that it is not typically a diagnosis that an individual would receive as it is understood as a symptomatic condition that presents itself in other diseases, and therefore a diagnosis may not be present. More likely, an individual would be diagnosed with PCOS with features of androgen excess. According to the literature, the majority of individuals with hyperandrogenism will have PCOS (Yildiz 167). The problem for me became finding a recruitment solution where I could speak to potential participants in a way they understood, while at the same time recruiting individuals who were eligible.

I chose to move forward with a symptom criterion list. It was detailed in information provided to the participants, including within the consent form, that to be eligible for the study, participants must have the ability to speak and write in English, be 18 years old or over, self-identify as having hyperandrogenism, and have experienced two or more of the symptoms of PCOS. Participants must have experienced one symptom from List A and at least one other symptom from List B which is not the same symptom as List A. List A includes symptoms of hyperandrogenism, such as excess body and facial hair and male-pattern-baldness. The symptoms of List B include all symptoms of hyperandrogenism plus additional non-androgen-excess symptoms of PCOS such as insulin resistance and Type 2 diabetes. This slightly complex criterion was necessary because it allowed for the inclusion of participants who were experiencing at least two symptoms of PCOS, with at least one of those symptoms "threatening" normative femininity. This eligibility requirement would exclude, for example, a participant who has PCOS and is experiencing high blood pressure and diabetes, exclusively. In this example, the participant with PCOS might not reflect on issues of gendered embodiment in their illness narrative.

A two PCOS symptom threshold was chosen to simplify the eligibility markers to ensure potential participants who have lived experience with hyperandrogenism could be included in the study. Most of the symptoms included on List A, and many on List B, encompass recognizing a change in secondary-sex characteristics rather than data from a medical test result. Further, a two-symptom threshold for diagnosis mirrors the clinical diagnosis of PCOS, notably lacking the same nuance and specific symptoms. Due to the complexity of PCOS and hyperandrogenism, both do not have universal diagnostic recommendations. Health care providers may take several approaches to diagnose PCOS that may include a combination of pelvic exams, hormonal blood tests and ultrasounds. Many times, a diagnostic method called the Rotterdam consensus may be used which defines PCOS "by the presence of two of three of the following criteria: oligo-anovulation, hyperandrogenism and polycystic ovaries (≥ 12 follicles measuring 2–9 mm in diameter and/or an ovarian volume > 10 mL in at least one ovary)" (Smet and McLennan 59). In a clinical setting, this may look like a patient being identified as having two of the three experiences: irregular or infrequent periods, a blood test or clinical signs of elevated androgens, and/or a scan showing polycystic ovaries. Clinical signs of elevated androgens indicate a presence of hyperandrogenism and are typically noted as the visual presence of hirsutism determined by using a standardized face and body hair growth scoring system (Yildiz 167). Maintaining lived experience with two symptoms as a threshold for participation acted as a method to circumvent, to an extent, this diagnostic gatekeeping.

Upon receiving an email from a potential participant expressing interest, an informational email was sent in response which detailed the study's objectives, process, participation expectations and eligibility requirements. Over the course of recruitment, more than fifty individuals requested further information. Those who confirmed their eligibility and willingness to participate were invited to a short screening interview conducted over Zoom. The interview included three sections: an informational preamble, an eligibility check and a diversity questionnaire. Participants were informed of their right to end the interview at any time, to pass on any question they found uncomfortable, and that while audio and video were not recorded, responses would be documented in a survey form. The eligibility section was critical to ensure that participants met the study's criteria, while the diversity section gathered demographic and identity-related information, including gender identity, sexuality, ethnicity, disability status, age, residence, body size, body image concerns and experience with autobiographical writing. Participants were explicitly reminded that this section was voluntary and that their responses, if given, would be used to explore how identity shapes and is shaped by hyperandrogenism without being linked back to them personally.

The screening interview was designed in a way to enhance the capability of producing qualitative responses that centred lived experience. Although many answers were outlined as checkboxes, there was an effort to include a multitude of options, prompting questions and space for nuanced notes. Further, lived experience was prioritized through language such as "do you consider yourself to be…, "have you ever experienced…," and "how would you describe…" As detailed in Chapter 2, an effort was made in each screening interview to convey small moments of my own experience with hyperandrogenism in order to establish a connection and to implicate myself as the researcher in the research process. Table 4.1 demonstrates the participant pool makeup in relation to the screening interview markers.

Fourteen eligible participants signed the consent form after reviewing the study's purpose, expectations, and data protection measures. They were given access to the *Click Me* Twine Writing Module, which they could complete at their own pace, though participation varied, with only ten ultimately finishing the module. Four participants did not complete it and did not respond to follow-up emails, and it was assumed that they were no longer interested. The module design phase involved developing a Twine illness narrative module, *Click Me*, which was created using Twine and published on itch.io, a platform for hosting indie video games. This platform was

*Table 4.1* Participant Identity Markers. Self-Reported Participant Identity Markers Collected in Screening Interviews of *Click Me* Study

| *Residence* | | *Age* | | *Person of Colour, a Racialized Person, or Mixed Race* | | *Aboriginal, First Nations, Métis, Inuit, or Indigenous Person* | |
|---|---|---|---|---|---|---|---|
| Canada | 8 | 20s | 6 | Yes | 5 | Yes | 1 |
| USA | 2 | 30s | 4 | No | 5 | No | 9 |
| *Disabled Person or Person with a Disability* | | *Body Size* | | *Experienced Body Image Concerns Around Not Feeling Feminine Enough* | | *Gender Identity* | |
| Yes | 2 | Average or Thin | 6 | Yes | 8 | Cis/Female/Woman | 9 |
| No | 8 | Plus | 4 | No | 2 | Nonbinary | 1 |
| *Sexual Orientation* | | *Received Healthcare Treatment or Visited a Healthcare Facility for Symptoms of Hyperandrogenism* | | *Psychiatric Disability or Mental Health Issues* | | *Prior Experience Writing About Living with Hyperandrogenism* | |
| Heterosexual/Straight | 5 | Yes | 10 | Yes | 5 | Yes | 5 |
| Queer Identity | 5 | No | 0 | No | 5 | No | 5 |

chosen over traditional file hosting services like Google Drive because it avoids compromising the technical features of the Twine module. The module featured images, sounds and interactive elements, designed with the 1980s arcade game aesthetic to evoke a Web 1.0 nostalgia and telegraph the use of hypertext in gameplay. The design incorporated computer code, a neon colour scheme reminiscent of arcade lights, and free-sourced arcade melodies that aligned with key climactic moments. Prior to participant use, the module was informally beta-tested to address technical bugs and design flaws, and at the time of the study, participants accessed it through the Twine 2.3.8 release in the Harlowe 3.1.0 story format.

After completing the *Click Me* module and uploading their Twine stories, ten authors participated in a closing interview to discuss their experience writing an illness narrative. The insight from these encounters will be detailed in-depth in later chapters of this book. From here, authors were given the option to share their Twine stories in a communal, secure folder that other *Click Me* authors had access to. This process was set up to speak to the community-building aspect of illness narratives. All ten authors submitted their stories to the communal drive. Participants were informed that the portal would be open for one month. They were also advised to permanently delete any Twine story files that they downloaded to their personal computers.

Finally, after successfully receiving a research grant, authors were each given a fifty dollar in-kind reward in the form of a gift card for their participation. In this study, I am working with underrepresented groups. Through diversity markers in screening interviews, I understand that all of the *Click Me* authors identify as a marginalized identity (a Person of Colour, Indigenous, a person with a psychiatric or physical disability, Queer gender identity and/or Queer sexual orientation). Reflecting on feminist research methods scholarship (Warnock et al. 195) about compensating underrepresented groups for their labour and time in research, I concluded that an in-kind reward was appropriate. In thinking critically about how compensation affects consent, I chose to recruit participants without advertising an in-kind reward in order to connect with participants who were interested in volunteering their time to advance research on hyperandrogenism. The in-kind reward was offered to authors at the completion of the study.

The final stage of the *Click Me* research was the data analysis phase. Data in the form of the anonymized Twine stories and the closing interview transcripts were coded first thematically using the NVivo qualitative coding software. The data in this project required a methodology that could examine how narrativity creates meaning through digital technology. One of the major projects of this research involved the development of a unique critical discourse analysis for digital-born narrative (CDADN). CDADN amalgamates important aspects of critical discourse analysis with some aspects of narrative analysis, digital discourse analysis, critical code studies and feminist new materialist theory, to produce a methodology that examines the discursive power dynamics and materiality of narratives online. This CDADN adopts a macro-social meaning of "narrative" defined by Ruth Page in her 2018 book *Narratives Online* as "not specific, verbal accounts of a particular set of events, but rather a general way of describing events or patterns of social-cultural behavior" (5–6). This is an important note as Page's definition allows for a honing of the concept of digital narratives as a network that includes all variations of the *Click Me* data. The research data includes not only the Twine narratives authors have submitted but also interview transcripts, screenshots of the visual interface of the Twines, code, images included in the Twines, and hypertexts. These differing forms of data fail to be comprehensively captured in Page's definition of narrative, however, they become extensions or components of digital narrative and therefore, I argue, can be captured in a methodological analysis of digital-born narratives, in this way. In other words, CDADN is a methodology that centres digital-born narratives at the root of the corpus but invites differing forms of data that may emerge to be analyzed in relation to the narrative.

## *Click Me* Twine Module Design

In the first stage of research for this project, I developed a Twine module to support the facilitation of writing illness narratives in literary hypertext. The *Click Me* Twine module was designed using some perspectives of narrative therapy, in particular the work of Renee Dumaresque, Taylor Thornton, Daniela Glaser and Anthony Lawrence in their article "Politicized Narrative Therapy" which uses anti-colonial discursive frameworks, critical race theory and counter-storytelling, Black feminist thought, and anti-sanist theorizing to reimagine narrative therapy as a means to enact political change. Dumaresque et al.'s political framing of narrative therapy was chosen as a framework to inform the development of the Twine module because of its affinity with Martinez and Fleck-Henderson's notion of health liberation (as discussed in Chapter 1). Health liberation, and in this context political narrative therapy, positions illness as a social justice issue rather than an individualized aliment and turns to social, institutional and political-based solutions.

Akin to illness narratives' sociohistorical identity as a political tool of counter-practice to normative medical approaches to healing, "Politicized Narrative Therapy" argues that traditional approaches to narrative therapy are deeply saturated in colonial perspectives that uphold neoliberal foundations in healthcare (Dumaresque et al. 109). The authors work to situate the practice of narrative therapy within a neoliberal desire to commodify recovery as an economy of therapy which sees illness narratives taken up as marketing content. Within this structure, the work of getting well becomes the responsibility and financial burden of the individual and this upholds the psychiatric institution as an authority (Dumaresque et al. 109). The authors argue that narrative therapy, "born from the intersection of whiteness and social work" (Dumaresque et al. 111), has a legacy rooted deeply in Eurocentric origins and engagement with this framework must be concerned with the ways in which perspectives of Indigenous and racialized cultures become legitimized through their co-option by formal psychiatry and medicine (Dumaresque et al. 113). The *Click Me* project is concerned with repositioning hyperandrogenism as a political identity and therefore it became important for the framework used to develop the therapeutic perspectives of the module to reflect this. Dumaresque et al. offer a four-step framework for politicizing the practice of narrative therapy, by which the design of the *Click Me* Twine module, closing interviews and community-building portal were informed.

According to Dumaresque et al., the practice of narrative therapy emerged from a desire to resist traditional methods and approaches to medicine, such as a biomedical model that pathologized emotional distress as an ailment of the body. Informed by Foucault's conceptualization of discourse and power as constructive and productive, narrative therapy, in theory, understands language as a political agent and the ways in which people narrativize their lives works to shape experiences of reality. As Dumaresque et al. describe "Knowledge created by bodies in power results in taken-for-granted truth claims that discredit, displace, and silence subjugated knowledges, producing norms, defining deviance, and therefore governing lives" (Dumaresque et al. 115). In the process of externalization of narrative in narrative therapy, Dumaresque et al. argue that while some therapists appropriately work to support the flourishing of alternative truths that challenge oppressive knowledge systems, many fail to effectively deconstruct or intervene in the insuperable nature of dominant discourse (116).

Dumaresque et al. give the example of therapists who treat neurodiverse children. When a narrative therapy approach fails to call into question the mechanics of diagnosis, "therapists are complicit in reinforcing the violence inherent in the medical model" (Dumaresque et al. 116). Yet, beyond complacency, therapy professionals are offered limited resources in the biomedical model that may work to challenge ineffective approaches to supporting the well-being of the patient (Dumaresque et al. 116). The research question at the core of the *Click Me* work intentionally avoids veering into the realm of a formal medical-therapeutic inquiry. It does not ask about measurable outcomes regarding mental health questionnaires and/or reduction of symptoms (although these factors are significant and valuable). By asking about the development of positive relationships between the self and world, the *Click Me* research question is attempting to grapple with meaning made from the intersection of the individual with the structural–political in a way that foregrounds the individual's experiences with systems, structures and institutions that may participate in the pathologizing of their identity. Dumaresque et al.'s interpretation of narrative therapy offers the *Click Me* research generative methods to frame the process of illness narrative authorship not as an individualized treatment method, but as a political act.

The initial step in the process of narrative therapy is to identify the problem story or an unhelpful sense of reality that a person may hold about themselves (Dumaresque et al. 118). In a typical approach to the method, a therapist may engage with the patient to identify the problem story and then work to challenge the inherent assumptions that uphold it. Dumaresque et al. argue, though, that the act of destabilizing the problem story must go further to make visible the dominant discourses that underpin this story and become the foundation of our belief systems. This is the process of connecting the problem story to larger sociocultural, historical, and political contexts (Dumaresque et al. 118). For the *Click Me* module, it became important that an identification of the problem story relating to the experience of hyperandrogenism as a political identity had to be unearthed prior to the authors writing their illness narratives. This was because, although all authors in screening interviews framed their illness to me in a way that acknowledged their experience as political, I wanted to ensure that each author understood the sociohistorical context. This was done through several choices made throughout the module.

The *Click Me* module is divided into six parts with the second section devoted to the topic of hyperandrogenism. The *Click Me* authors read passages that describe a clinical description of the illness as well as common symptoms that can arise. Authors are then prompted to think about the distress many individuals with hyperandrogenism experience, not only from the physical manifestations of the disease but also from perceptions of failing to meet a particular standard of womanhood. The rest of the section focuses on the story of Caster Semenya, a South African Olympic track runner who was mandated by the IAAF to undergo a "sex-verification" test following a public inquiry into her biological sex. As described in depth in Chapter 2, the IAAF ruled that Semenya had to pharmaceutically lower her natural levels of testosterone in order to compete in the women's category of her sport. In the telling of Semenya's story, authors click through passages that describe Semenya's public reflections on the injustice of her experiences, as shown in Figure 4.1, and further context into how the IAAF facilitates bans on particular bodies over others. Near the end of this section of the module, the authors read a passage that outlines several assumptions that underpin the IAAF's decision, including that biological sex is a binary where there are only male and female bodies, athletic competitions are already level playing fields for those who compete, and high testosterone always gives an athletic advantage (Savulescu). Rather than overtly challenge these beliefs, the module invites the author to consider: "what do you think?" This moment of

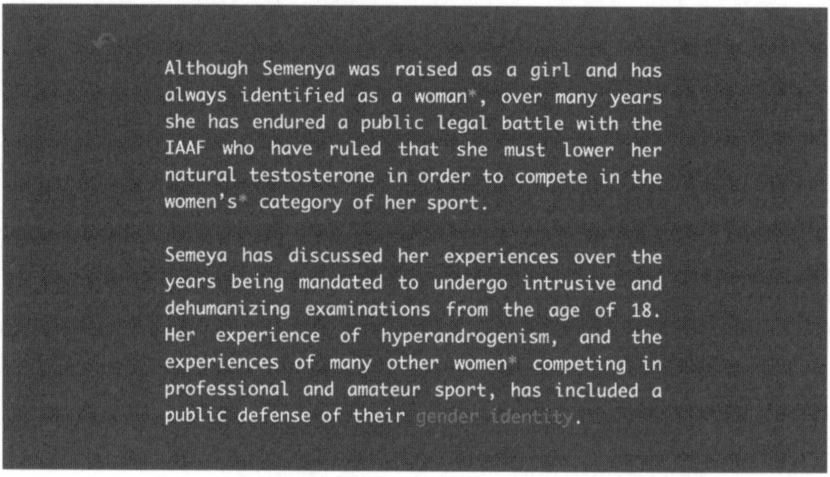


*Figure 4.1* Screenshot A of Twine Illness Narrative Module.

reflection opens space for the author to engage with the information provided by the module in relation to their own experience with hyperandrogenism to perhaps connect their experience to Semenya's.

It is important to locate the problem story within the sociocultural context, as through the experience of Caster Semenya, however, it is equally vital to identify the problem discourse within the author's individualized reality. In part three of the module, authors were led through a storyboarding exercise that later became the foundation for their Twine illness narrative. The *Click Me* authors are asked to reflect on the moments that have defined their illness experience. As brief or descriptive as they prefer, authors are asked to write down, on a piece of paper, three titles that represent three of the most important moments of their illness. For each moment, authors are invited to choose a colour to represent how they felt in that moment, along with descriptions of what that colour represents to them.[1] At this point in the module, authors engage in a seven-minute, low-stakes free writing exercise. The *Click Me* module explains that free writing is a technique for building narratives where the author writes about a topic continuously for a set amount of time. What is important for free writing is that thoughts about grammar, spelling, or punctuation should refrain from impeding the flow of writing. The authors are encouraged to use their "moments" as a home base to build their narratives and are offered different options for connecting with one, two or all three of their moments.

Figure 4.2 shows the free writing passage with the following writing prompt that centres embodiment: "In this Moment, how did it *feel* to be in

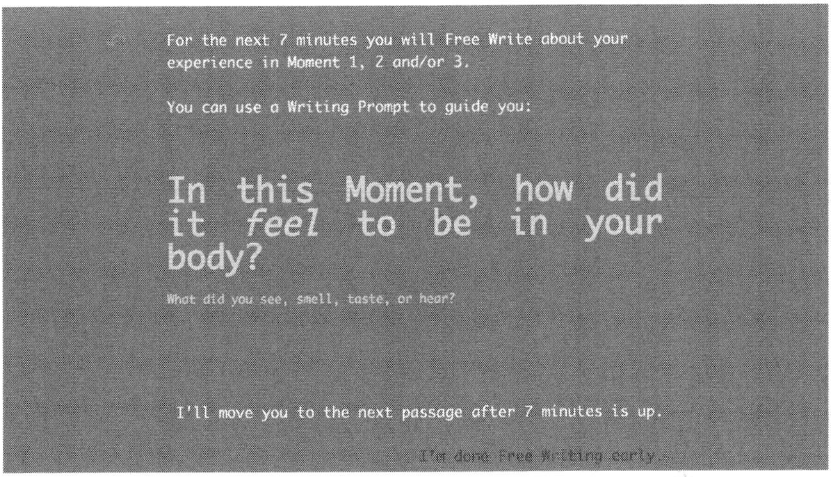


*Figure 4.2* Screenshot B of Twine Illness Narrative Module.

your body? What did you see, smell, taste, or hear?" This passage is set on a seven-minute timer and plays instrumental music in the background which authors are given the option to silence. The choice to offer background music during Twine writing exercises was informed by feedback from author workshops for a related research project I contributed to, *Writing New Bodies* (Ensslin et al.), introduced in Chapter 1 of this book. The authors in *Writing New Bodies* suggested a popular YouTube stream which was used in the *Click Me* Twine module for this study. Following the encouragement of a break to respond to physical or emotional needs brought up during the free writing process, authors are asked to complete the final step of storyboarding their narratives.

Authors are then asked to brainstorm a list of themes that may thread through each of their three defining moments. Here, they encounter a passage that provides some example themes that may be a helpful starting point, such as control, body positivity and social media. The author is now shown a passage that reads: "Your paper may look something like this." Below the text is an example of what an author's paper may look similar to at this final stage (Figure 4.3). This closes the third part of the module and authors are encouraged to use this exercise as the foundation for their Twine illness narrative if they choose. The practice of storyboarding the illness narrative, at this stage of the module, is an effort to identify the problem story and dominant discourse by pulling out the embodied experience of the author in the wake of engaging with the political context of the disease.

In typical approaches to narrative therapy, the second step in the therapeutic process is to externalize the problem story. According to Dumaresque et al., externalizing work is a direct response to what narrative therapists

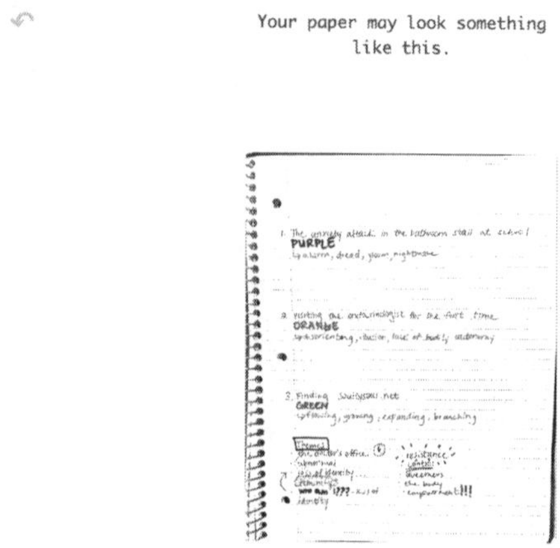


*Figure 4.3* Screenshot C of Twine Illness Narrative Module.

believe is a chronic internalizing by the patient (119). This manoeuver to unify the individual with the problem story makes it difficult to connect experiences to the larger sociopolitical context and understand the systems of power that contribute to upholding the structure of the problem story. Dumaresque et al. call these "totalizing self-narratives" and argue that they often cause individuals to "experience feelings that negatively impact their life, such as blame, guilt, and isolation" (119). The process of externalizing the problem story starts by identifying how, when and where the issue affects the patient's life and then turns to exploring how it has persisted over time (Dumaresque et al. 120). Then, the therapist and the patient collectively agree on a label to name the problem. This act works to identify the problem story as an entity separate from the self. However, Dumaresque et al. push this practice further through a call to not only externalize the problem story but to politicize it. The authors argue that the act of identifying the problem story and removing it from the internal self fails to dislodge the larger socio-structural factors that may have situated the problem story as a political experience of oppression.

As described in Chapter 1, the use of gendered language is complex in this project. Hyperandrogenism is a deeply gender-saturated illness where clinical diagnosis is reliant on understanding an incongruence between biological sex and embodiment. It is critical to speak about these gendered implications, however, *Click Me* authors and individuals diagnosed with the disease are not only women. One of the initial acts of externalization taken in the Twine module was attempting to destabilize the relationship between the individual and their gender identity. This was not an attempt to claim

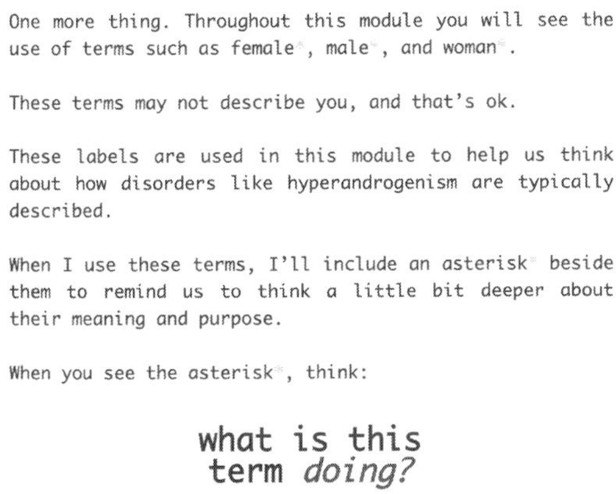


*Figure 4.4* Screenshot D of Twine Illness Narrative Module.

that gender identity is somehow not inherent to our sense of self, however, it was important to have authors look at the concept of womanhood as outside of themselves so they may have a vantage point to interrogate its presumed coherence. Figure 4.4 shows a passage that appears during the instructional section of the module. The passage explains that gendered and sexed terms will be used throughout the module, but that they may not reflect the identity or experience of every author. During every instance of gendered and sexed language throughout the module, authors will see a flashing yellow asterisk beside the word. This feature is intended to remind the author to take up an externalized vantage point to think deeply about what function that term is performing.

As the *Click Me* module progresses, a passage details several of the many symptoms that hyperandrogenism is linked to, followed by the note: "Dealing with any of these symptoms is scary because we live in a culture that sets high standards for what it means to be a woman*." The flashing asterisk beside the term *woman*, here, is intended to encourage the author to reflect, not only on what these high standards may be but what being a woman might mean to them. Authors are led through a series of passages that grapple with some basic stereotypes of womanhood that hyperandrogenism disrupts. One passage asks authors to choose how to complete the sentence: "Women* are always:" with hyperlinked terms such as [[Thin]], [[Demure]], [[Hairless]], [[Fertile]], or—off kilter and offset on its own line—the word [[Healthy]]. When the author chooses one of these options, they are brought to a jarring passage with red letters that challenges the author to consider: "Are They?" This passage sequence is intended to invite the author to engage with a gendered stereotype, and then pause them in a passage to question these assumptions.

Once the author chooses the hypertext "[[Healthy]]" the next passage asks the reader to consider: "What does it mean to you to be healthy?" This moment is designed to position the author to think about binaries such as *health* and *illness* and how hyperandrogenism fits into that narrative. For example, an author might consider, here, that they may have internalized beliefs that a hairless body means a healthy body. Ideally, the author has an opportunity here to reflect on the distress that hyperandrogenism embodiment causes and make a link to any internalized assumptions around gender expression that may contribute to this distress. This is a small moment to begin to shift the distress from an internal failure to meet standards of gender to the external cultural expectations of how the body should present.

One of the most critical aspects of this project is grappling with the experience of individuals with hyperandrogenism in the normative healthcare system. Therefore, working to externalize distress around the patient-healthcare provider encounter and connect it to larger political contexts was important. During a section of the Twine module, authors are asked to reflect on how they may feel when they visit the doctor. A passage that explains how some individuals with hyperandrogenism have a difficult time when they visit the doctor, followed by a list of example reasons, including "They weren't listened to," "Their symptoms were dismissed," and "They weren't treated like a person." These examples are barely visible and only become legible once the author hovers their cursor over them, a design choice to convey a sense of revealing hidden notions of shame.

The module continues:

> It's almost impossible to block out all these messages that say something is wrong with your body. Some women* have even described their bodies as: Dysfunctional, abnormal, or sick. It isn't talked about very much, so hyperandrogenism can be lonely, too.

This section is followed by a passage that explains that many individuals deal with hyperandrogenism and some of them use writing as a method to cope with emotional distress. This section is intended to externalize and politicize negative experiences born from hyperandrogenism's contact with the healthcare system. If authors have felt dehumanized in their healthcare encounters, rather than situating themselves or their bodies as the problem origin, the module attempts to shift the narrative to challenge the system's capacity to appropriately respond to nuances of biological sex embodiment.

After the identification and externalization of the problem story, what follows in the narrative therapy process is typically the development of alternative, generative stories of the self. For the therapeutic process, identifying alternative stories begins first with interrogating the power of the problem. According to Dumaresque et al., narrative therapists might work with clients to identify moments, both historically and currently, where the problem lacked control over the individual, or the individual gained power over the problem (122). Mapping moments of agency for the individual, according to the authors, works to destabilize the perceived omnipotence of the problem as all-encompassing to the life of the individual. Dumaresque et al. refer to these moments of exception as "unique outcomes" and argue that these details can be used to construct an alternative narrative of the individual's experience (122). Individuals, here, can reimagine their identities, lives, and relationships free from the problem, allowing them to explore new and preferred ways of being.

In this process, narrative therapists might ask individuals to think deeply about their lives absent from the context of their dominant story, how it would look, and how they might feel. This enacts the process of re-authoring their dominant story in a way that opens up space to develop an alternative, productive narrative of the self. For Dumaresque et al., however, the reauthoring of the alternative story must also include the production of alternative discourses that challenge the dominant, restrictive ways of knowing that facilitate complex forms of oppression. The authors distinguish alternative stories as avenues for personal meaning-making, while alternative discourses challenge dominant narratives by centring marginalized knowledge and values (Dumaresque et al. 122). The authors use the case study of a "Latin American woman named Sofia" who was seeking therapy due to perceived feelings of "worthlessness" in her marriage. Sofia's dominant discourse of worthlessness was identified, externalized and reframed in a political way as domestic abuse and "white colonial patriarchy" (Dumaresque et al. 123). Sofia was led to identify moments where the dominant discourse of worthlessness may have been absent, such as during "community organizing with other women [which] made her acknowledge all of her skills, passion, and labour, which go unappreciated and undervalued in much of society and in her home" (Dumaresque et al. 123). Through this process of political narrative therapy, the practitioner was able to counter Sofia's initial self-loathing for a perceived inability to be a "good" wife and reframe the narrative in a way that the patient understood and embraced as race and gender-based oppression, reinforced through the abuse of her husband.

As discussed in Chapter 1, the *Click Me* Twine module was not intended to facilitate formal therapy, narrative or otherwise, for the *Click Me* authors. It stands as a tool for individuals to use to write illness narratives. There is no therapy professional guiding the writing process and the experience is intended to be accessed by individuals in isolation if needed. Therefore, the third step in Dumaresque et al.'s narrative therapy process is not directly implemented into the *Click Me* Twine module, however, there are moments and outcomes that do reflect the impact of reauthoring and alternative discourse formation. Most notably, authors appeared to have engaged with the processes of alternative story building in the writing of their Twine illness narratives, which will be discussed in later chapters of this book.

In the final section of the module, authors are invited to write their own illness narrative in Twine based on their experience with hyperandrogenism. The *Click Me* authors are instructed to think deeply about what story they desire to tell. The illness narratives can be new or an expanded version of the storyboarding exercise, but critically, the module notes that there are no expectations for this piece of work and authors are free to build their story the way that feels right to them. Authors are reminded: "You are the author. Your story can be long, or very short. Don't worry about writing a 'perfect' or even 'finished' piece of work, instead, focus on reflecting on your memories in a new way." Once the author is ready to write, they click the hypertext that brings them to a new writing prompt: "What is it like to live in a body with hyperandrogenism?" The writing process of the module is designed to take around 45 minutes, however, authors are able to use the amount of time they prefer. The writing prompt passage includes a list of hypertexts to remind authors of the technical aspects of Twine detailed in earlier sections of the module. This passage is coded with sound-adjustable instrumental music and a timer of 45 minutes. The module brings the author to the next passage when the time runs out, but authors are able to leave the passage early or return to it afterwards.

An additional and critical opportunity to engage with the process of alternative discourse writing was during the closing interview of the study. The closing interview was intentionally brief and open-ended, consisting of two questions, with various prompts to expand responses. The first question asks what the author's experience was using Twine and the second how the author might describe their feelings towards their body, identity, or ideas about where they fit in the world after writing about their illness. The second question includes a caveat that this may look like having a new, positive perspective on how the body is perceived in the world or perhaps developing a kinder evaluation of the body. The first open-ended question of the interview is intended to gather information and feedback on the accessibility and usability of Twine as a tool. This speaks to understanding, beyond the therapeutic value of illness narratives, the feasibility of the technical aspects of the method as enabling or inhibiting the writing process (or, likely, a combination of both). The second question seeks to explore the therapeutic value and contribution to a more generative relationship to the self, facilitated through the writing process. Both questions, in relation to one another, seek to answer the research question of this study: how can women and nonbinary individuals with hyperandrogenism use literary hypertext technology to write illness narratives that construct positive relationships between their identities and the world? In this sense, how can positive relationships be constructed both through the therapeutic and technical process of writing literary hypertext?

The final step in Dumaresque et al.'s political approach to narrative therapy is what the authors refer to as "thickening the thread" of the alternative story (124). In narrative therapy, this process typically involves reinforcing the alternative narrative through strategies such as artistic expression, support groups and deeper engagement with insights gained in therapy (Dumaresque et al. 124). The political reimaging of narrative therapy's thickening of the thread, for Dumaresque et al., is the act of establishing the alternative discourse as a collective narrative. Dumaresque et al. argue that rather than halting at the reinforcement of the alternative narrative, individual experiences of oppression should be linked to broader communities facing similar struggles (124). This is a critical step in the process to understand the alternative discourse as a sociohistorical actor that comes to shape not only the individual but also the community with which the individual identifies. The authors argue that if the biomedical model intends to treat the distress of the individual, healing and resistance must begin at the root of experience, or the community. This approach, according to the authors, will bring sustainable social change by positioning individualized distress as a responsibility for the larger collective.

The practice of thickening the thread and collectivizing experience that is central to political narrative therapy is similarly at the heart of the illness narrative genre. Locating a community through writing in the face of individualized subjugation, culturally and/or medically, has been a central way illness narratives have been taken up in scholarship. Finding a method to thicken the thread for this project, however, was complex. Protecting identities, respecting consent, and nourishing a safe space to share vulnerable stories were the highest priorities for conducting this research. Inserting the Twine illness narratives submitted by authors into a public online space where they could be mediated by communities of reader/players, theoretically, would speak to the essence of illness narratives as a community-building tool. However, this was not considered for this project for various reasons, including maintaining the anonymity of authors and shielding their personal stories from potential online discord.

Therefore, I decided to include a small-scale community-building aspect to the study where authors were invited to share their Twines in a secure and private folder for other *Click Me* authors to read. This was not a formal aspect of participation, and authors were informed that they were not required to share their stories. If they chose not to submit their Twines to the folder, their stories would still be included in the study. The community-building portal, to which all ten authors chose to contribute to, became one of the most vital aspects of the research process. The portal was open during the month of April 2021. As this was not a formal aspect of the study, authors were not interviewed about their experiences exploring the Twine stories of others, however, one author noted informally over email:

> I just spent the evening reading through everyone's story [sic] and I've been crying the entire time. I feel seen, heard and validated within my own experiences and feel a kinship with the other authors (even though they are anonymous).

This feedback from an author, who granted consent to publish this quote,, validates the intention of health liberation and thickening the thread of the illness experience, in the *Click Me* study and beyond.

At the heels of this module tutorial, to sing Twine's accessibility praises would be quite empty without acknowledging its stark limitations. The *Click Me* authors actually do this themselves, particularly bringing forward the concept of capacity in narrative authorship. More on that to come in subsequent chapters, however, in the design of this tutorial I want to state the obvious: Twine is a digital tool that requires an amount of digital literacy and physical connection to the internet to access. Therefore, the *Click Me* Twine module was not comprehensively accessible, for several reasons. First, participation in the study, and accessing Twine as an individual, requires access to a digital device and internet browser which is a limiting requirement. This leads to important questions surrounding tethers between marginalization and lack of digital access as well as age-related barriers. As discussed in earlier sections of this chapter, all of the *Click Me* authors could be considered relatively young. There was an evident absence of representation from older individuals with hyperandrogenism, and, as I mentioned above, this requires more information to understand if this outcome is because of potential struggles in adopting new technologies or perhaps because younger individuals are prone to seek out avenues to respond to their sex-based illness. Ultimately, I lack enough information to have the answer to this question.

Second, the *Click Me* module relied heavily on colour distinction in order to navigate through passages which may be a barrier for certain users, particularly those with colour vision deficiency. Although stark colour contrast was implemented through most of the module, tending to contrast ratios was not consistently carried out which may have impacted readability (in some passages the dark purple hypertexts are on a light purple background). Third, sounds were incorporated throughout the module, but these were intentionally included to supplement the experience and were not imperative for the completion of the exercises. Finally, and critically, Twine stories are not inherently accessible through all screen readers and have to be manipulated through intentional technical design and story format choices made by the author to ensure accessibility for various technologies. This is a significant issue when using Twine, or other literary hypertext software, as a teaching tool for groups of individuals who may need differing forms of access.

## Teaching Twine

In addition to design elements of the module that engage with the process of narrative building and the political framing of pathology, the module also had to stand as a pedagogical tool for the Twine technology. Building a comprehensive tutorial for new authors of literary hypertext was complex. Having the authors complete their Twine stories alone, in the privacy of their own space, was an intentional choice to reflect the identity of illness narratives as counter-practice to established medical institutions. This counter-practice has assumed a culture of speaking back to normative medicalized discourses where, oftentimes, an author's only act of resistance might be their individualized writing process. Therefore, it was important for the *Click Me* module to embody an understanding of this sociohistorical context and stand as a comprehensive resource. In order to accomplish this, the module was designed with six various sections including an introduction, a political framing of hyperandrogenism, an introduction to Twinery.org, storyboarding, a Twine tutorial, and the final illness narrative prompt. Several of these sections have been discussed above in the context of their relationship with narrative therapy.

This section will discuss the design of the technical instructive sections of the module as a pedagogical tool for teaching literary hypertext and the Twine technology. Much of the technical instructions of this module were heavily informed by feedback from the informal beta-testers of the module. As the majority of *Click Me* authors had no previous experience with literary hypertext, it was critical that the opening passages of the module include a linear and explicit navigation path, rather than rhizomatic, branching options that could have the potential to confuse a new reader/player. However, it was even more imperative that the module resisted making assumptions about an author's previous knowledge of the functionality of hypertext. I did not want to assume that authors would inherently be familiar with even typical displays of hypertext, such as a body of black text that includes a distinctly coloured, underlined word. The opening passages of the module, therefore, set the foundation for understanding where to click to move forward and through the exercise.

The module opens with a blinking hypertext that reads: "Click Me." This becomes the first indication that clicking certain text in the module will bring you to a new passage. Once the author clicks the text, they are brought to a

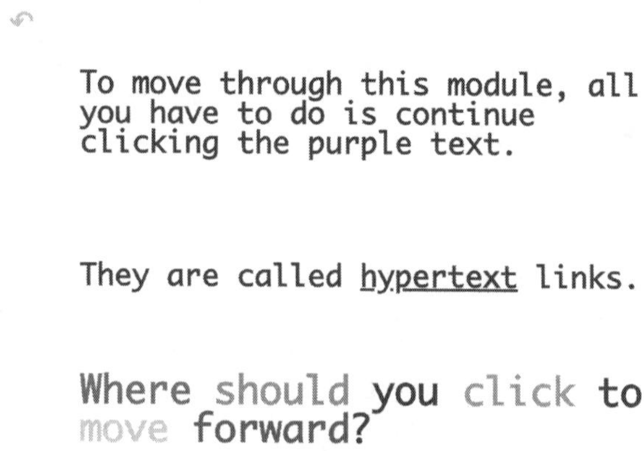


*Figure 4.5* Screenshot E of Twine Illness Narrative Module.

passage that reads: "Congrats! You navigated your first Twine passage!" The hypertext in this second passage is intentionally discernable and reads: "Next." However, not all the hypertexts in this module are intuitive in this way. Feedback from informal beta-testers noted that hypertext must be marked in a specific and uniform way that is obvious to the user who is navigating the module. The evident solution was to colour code the hypertext and make this known to the author. Although this method was successful with the authors in this study, future research should consider accessibility in relation to hypertext colour.

Figure 4.5 shows a passage explaining the colour code and ensures that authors understand this code before they move forward in the module. This passage contains various red herrings in the form of different coloured text and text marked in other ways that authors may recognize as hypertexts (e.g., underlined text and blinking text). Authors must click the word "Forward," which is in purple text, to move to the next passage. Finally, informal beta-testing noted that it was not intuitive that you may have to scroll down in the module to find the purple hypertexts. Therefore, the next passage of the module explains this feature: "Here's a tip: sometimes you might have to scroll down to find the purple hypertext links!" Once the author scrolls down on this page, they find a small hypertext that reads: "You found me!" In beta-testing, these instructional passages proved to be sufficient to effectively convey the nature of literary hypertext navigation.

It was critical for the *Click Me* module to be designed in a way that showcases how dynamic Twine stories can be and also the tool's identity as an interactive and rhizomatic storytelling technology. Through various coding elements, I built in interactive features that allowed authors to input certain information about themselves. For example, in one of the introductory passages, authors are asked to write their names into a text field. After this information is inputted, this data is inserted throughout the module into different sections to create a sense of a personalized experience for the author. In addition to a more connected experience, this passage is intended to display how Twine can incorporate interactive elements.

In order for *Click Me* authors to receive more robust encounters with Twine's interactive capabilities beyond what was possible in the module, it was important to connect them to a variety of dynamic published Twines. In the section that introduces authors to the Twine technology, they are invited to spend fifteen minutes reading/playing through at least two different Twine games. Here, the authors encounter a passage that provides links to seven different game options, including Anna Anthropy's *Queers in Love at the End of the World* and Zoë Quinn's *Depression Quest*. The module explains that some Twines are more complex than others, but not to let that discourage them as by the end of the module they will have all the tools required to build a simple story themselves. Following this exercise, the module explains that the intention of engaging with other Twine stories is to reveal how multifaceted the medium can be, noting: "funny, sad, shocking, autobiographical, make-believe, science fiction, disorientating…You Decide." While the majority of authors were new to literary hypertext and programming, and this module did not focus on skills for building complex aspects of Twine found in many of the stories authors read, there was an intention to embolden the authors to think deeply about what their stories can do.

Understanding the capacity for multiplicity in the Twine story structure was a key learning outcome of the module. The module itself was not rhizomatic in that it produced an identical user path for all *Click Me* authors. This was a critical design choice to ensure every author received the same information in their experience of the module. However, there were moments of rhizomatic multiplicity built into two separate sections. The first section is a scene with a simple A versus B hypertext path choice. A passage explains that Twine can build nonlinear stories and "by nonlinear, I'll show you what I mean." The following passage is marked by the clicking sound of a typewriter. Soon text begins to appear, letter by letter, writing the beginning of a familiar story. The passage reads: "Once upon a time… [Name pulled from interactive input] was walking through the woods. Suddenly they come across a fork in the path ahead." As shown in Figure 4.6, the author is asked to choose a direction to turn: right or left. Either hypertext can be chosen or this is the first moment in the module that displays a multiple path choice. If the author chooses left, they are confronted with a loud snap of thunder and subsequent sounds of rainfall. A dark image of a forest in a storm appears on the screen. The text explains that the storm is raging, and the forest path

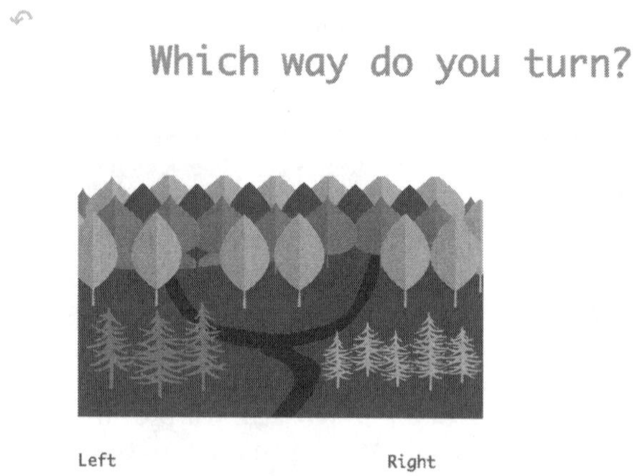


*Figure 4.6* Screenshot F of Twine Illness Narrative Module.

begins to flood at their feet. The passage probes: "Turn around and go right." Once the author chooses the right option, they hear birds chirping and are shown a sunny forest landscape accompanied by text that describes a warm and pleasant stroll as they eat raspberries from a bush. If the author chooses the right direction initially, the experience would be the same, but inverted. This is a basic, binary and oppositional structure for displaying choice in the narrative path that the authors can build into their own stories. The final passage in this section notes that "Building stories in Twine can be about choice. Where do you want your story to go?" Ultimately, this simple navigational exercise is intended to demonstrate the concept of a rhizomatic, multiple path narrative plot that authors may utilize in their own stories.

This navigational tutorial is supplemented later on in the *Click Me* module during the Twine tutorial section where *Click Me* authors are given an outline for three story path options, which I call a *forward path*, a *weaving path* and *multiple paths*. A forward path is when the story moves the reader/player through a straight line. The *Click Me* module is an example of a mainly forward path where the intention is to cultivate a uniform experience for every reader/player of the Twine. A weaving path branches the narrative into two or multiple hypertext passages but ultimately comes back to a single path. The final narrative structure, multiple paths, incorporates a multitude of hypertext paths for the reader/player to follow. In this structure, each path may describe a different plot and narrative conclusion. The module explains that multiple paths may be more complex and time-consuming to build, but they have the potential to be a generative method to "play through" different scenarios or dream up alternative ways things could have been in relation to

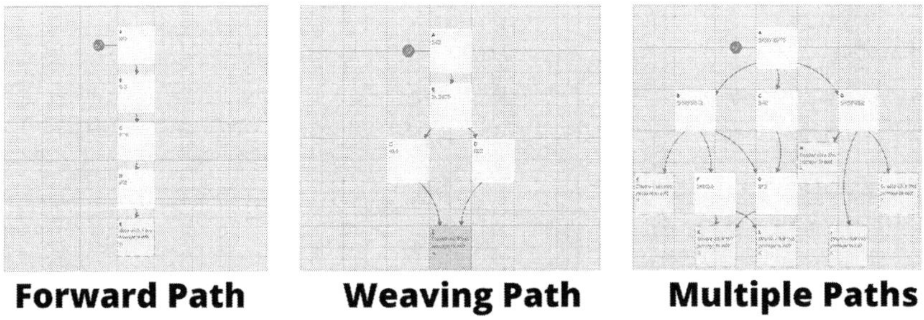


*Figure 4.7* Screenshot G of Twine Illness Narrative Module.

illness experience. Figure 4.7 shows example screenshots of what the Twine backend may look like following each story structure. The module explains that authors have the option to build their stories using any structure they prefer. Subsequent chapters will discuss what story structure was utilized most by the *Click Me* authors and the potential reasons for this.

Before authors encountered their final writing prompt to build their illness narratives, the module led them through a comprehensive Twine instructional tutorial. This section opens with a passage explaining the process of the tutorial, the expected outcomes for the author, and further resources for support including the popular Twine Wiki resource (Twine Wiki has retired at the end of 2020 and rolled into the Twine Cookbook). The *Click Me* authors are then taken through an eight-step tutorial on how to access and set up Twine from scratch, including how to access Twine in the browser, set up a new story, and name a new Twine file. The *Click Me* authors encounter a passage that shows the final step in this section which is describing how authors can change the story format of their Twine. The *Click Me* module instructs authors to select the Harlowe 3.1.0 version to ensure that the subsequent instructions in the module align for all authors. In the design process of the module, it was important that all textual instructions were supplemented by explicit visual cues to ensure that all authors felt confident moving through the module while producing their own work. I decided to include screenshots of the sections of the Twine interface the module was referring to, supplemented by stark red arrows and boxes to highlight the action. Each action that required the author to click on something was distinguished with the word "click" displayed in a turquoise text (HTML colour code [#69FFB9]) using a blinking feature ([text-style: "blink"] macro).

The remainder of the tutorial goes in-depth into how to write and publish a Twine story, including what a passage is, how to create an opening passage, how to test a story, what a hypertext is and how to code one (or more) hypertexts into a passage, how to create a linked passage through hypertext, saving a story, and leaving and returning to a work. Authors are also led through some basic codes that can be used to manipulate the style of the Twine including changing the colour of text and background, changing text features like italics and bold, and changing where the text appears on the screen (alignment). Following the comprehensive Twine tutorial, authors are led to the Twine illness narrative writing prompt discussed in a previous section of this chapter, where they have access to the Twine technical instructions through various hypertexts. Once the author completes their illness narrative, the module offers instructions on how to submit their file, thanks the author for their contribution and bravery, and details the next steps of the study.

Where the technical design choices and narrative therapy lens intersect, I believe, is in the ways in which the *Click Me* module is highly intentional in the path it guides the reader/player down, while at the same time allowing for open-ended experience. While the module was designed to carry out a linear path for all reader/players, the work it asks the authors to do is open to diverse expression. Authors are encouraged to build and design their stories of the self in ways that resonate with them—simple, grand, heartbreaking, clinical, littered with dead ends—ultimately, the choice is the authors' to make. The module ends with the note: "just because you're finished your Twine story, doesn't mean the story's over. How do you think the next chapter will go?"

## Note

1 Using colour association is one task-oriented approach for some methods of therapy for trauma treatment (Rankin and Taucher 140).

## Works Cited

Anthropy, Anna. *Queers in Love at the End of the World*. itch.io, 12 March 2016, https://w.itch.io/end-of-the-world

Dumaresque, Renee, et al. "Politicized Narrative Therapy: A Reckoning and a Call to Action." *Canadian Social Work Review/Revue Canadienne de Service Social*, vol. 35, no. 1, 2018, pp. 109–129.

Ensslin, Astrid, et al. *Writing New Bodies*. Project website, 2019, https://sites.google.com/ualberta.ca/writingnewbodies/home

Klimas, Chris. *Twine*. The Interactive Technology Foundation, 2009, http://twinery.org/

Martinez, Dawn Belkin, and Ann Fleck-Henderson. *Social Justice in Clinical Practice: A Liberation Health Framework for Social Work*. Routledge, 2014.

McGowan, Mary P. "Polycystic Ovary Syndrome: A Common Endocrine Disorder and Risk Factor for Vascular Disease." *Current Treatment Options in Cardiovascular Medicine*, vol. 13, no. 4, 2011, pp. 289–301.

Oakley, Amanda. "Hyperandrogenism." *DermNet NZ*, 2014, https://www.dermnetnz.org/topics/hyperandrogenism/. Accessed 19 February 2020.

Page, Ruth. *Narratives Online: Shared Stories in Social Media*. Cambridge University Press, 2018.

Quinn, Zoë. *Depression Quest*. The Quinnspiracy, 14 February 2013, http://www.depressionquest.com/

Rankin, Anita B. and Lindsay C. Taucher. "A Task-Oriented Approach to Art Therapy in Trauma Treatment." *Art Therapy*, vol. 20, no. 3, pp. 138–147.

Savulescu, Julian. "Ten Ethical Flaws in the Caster Semenya Decision on Intersex in Sport." *The Conversation*, 9 May 2019, https://theconversation.com/ten-ethical-flaws-in-the-caster-semenya-decision-on-intersex-in-sport-116448

Smet, Maria Elisabeth, McLennan, Andrew. "Rotterdam Criteria, The End." *Australasian Journal of Ultrasound in Medicine*, vol. 21, no. 2, 2018, pp. 59–60

*Twine Cookbook*. Twinery.org, 2021, https://twinery.org/cookbook/

"Twine Reference." Twine Documentation, *Twinery.org*, https://twinery.org/reference/en/. Accessed 25 March 2025.

Warnock, Rosalie, et al. "Should We Pay Research Participants? Feminist Political Economy for Ethical Practices in Precarious Times." *Area*, vol. 54, no. 2, 2022, pp. 195–202.

Yildiz, Bulent O. "Diagnosis of Hyperandrogenism: Clinical Criteria." *Best Practice & Research: Clinical Endocrinology & Metabolism*, vol. 20, no. 2, 2006, pp. 167–176.

# 5 The Abnormal Body

## Coding the Hypertext

Returning to the question at the centre of this book, I am reminded that my intention is to explore insight from both the technical aspects of hypertext software and thematic patterns in story worlds that may contribute to the development of positive relationship building for the *Click Me* authors. How can women and nonbinary individuals with hyperandrogenism use literary hypertext technology to write illness narratives that construct positive relationships between their identities and the world? The purpose of looking at hypertext's value is to open space for the inverse as well. Through this approach, analysis can situate aspects of the research that did not add value, did not contribute to positive relationship building or were perceived as inaccessible by the *Click Me* authors. This chapter will have dual intentions: analyze the research findings and discuss the meaning generated from those findings. This chapter looks at the common themes in the *Click Me* Twines, beginning with the discourse construction of the abnormal body. The chapter then turns to the relational aspects of the illness narratives by looking at how relationships between the author and their community shape, and both construct and deconstruct the *sick* identity. This chapter also analyzes narrative perspective and contemplates why each *Click Me* narrative used the first-person point of view to position the narrator. Finally, it provides insights into what is put forward or left out of the *Click Me* authors' framing of their Twine narratives and shows how authors mediate their stories with external texts and audiences.

Table 5.1 shows a list of Affect, Embodiment and Identity, Feminist New Materialist and Health-related codes and the frequency in which they were coded in the *Click Me* data using the software NVivo. The meta-category of Affect, Embodiment and Identity includes codes such as The Body, Shame and Resistance. It also includes parent codes that house child codes. For example, the parent code Family houses the child code Sister. Each time a *Click Me* Twine narrative referenced the topic of a sister, the text excerpt

DOI: 10.4324/9781003646921-5

*Table 5.1* Affect, Embodiment and Identity, Feminist New Materialist and Health-Related Code Frequency

| *Code* | *Number of Coding References* |
|---|---|
| Codes\\Health\Symptoms | 116 |
| Codes\\Health\Healthcare System | 95 |
| Codes\\Affect, Embodiment and Identity Themes\The Body | 71 |
| Codes\\Affect, Embodiment and Identity Themes\Change in Perspective | 47 |
| Codes\\Affect, Embodiment and Identity Themes\Connected Experiences | 33 |
| Codes\\Affect, Embodiment and Identity Themes\Identity | 32 |
| Codes\\Affect, Embodiment and Identity Themes\Unknown or Answer Seeking | 32 |
| Codes\\Affect, Embodiment and Identity Themes\Family\Mother | 28 |
| Codes\\Affect, Embodiment and Identity Themes\Relationships | 28 |
| Codes\\Feminist New Materialist Theory\Rhizome | 27 |
| Codes\\Affect, Embodiment and Identity Themes\Adolescence | 26 |
| Codes\\Affect, Embodiment and Identity Themes\Education and Knowledge Dissemination | 26 |
| Codes\\Affect, Embodiment and Identity Themes\Support | 25 |
| Codes\\Feminist New Materialist Theory\Difference | 24 |
| Codes\\Affect, Embodiment and Identity Themes\Empowerment | 23 |
| Codes\\Affect, Embodiment and Identity Themes\Femininity | 22 |
| Codes\\Feminist New Materialist Theory\Space | 21 |
| Codes\\Affect, Embodiment and Identity Themes\Reflection | 20 |
| Codes\\Feminist New Materialist Theory\Matter | 20 |
| Codes\\Affect, Embodiment and Identity Themes\Shame | 18 |
| Codes\\Feminist New Materialist Theory\Senses | 17 |
| Codes\\Affect, Embodiment and Identity Themes\Trauma | 15 |
| Codes\\Affect, Embodiment and Identity Themes\Abnormality | 14 |
| Codes\\Affect, Embodiment and Identity Themes\Family\Sister | 14 |
| Codes\\Feminist New Materialist Theory\Dualism (Complicating) | 13 |
| Codes\\Affect, Embodiment and Identity Themes\Control | 12 |

(*continued*)

*Table 5.1* (Continued)

| *Code* | *Number of Coding References* |
|---|---|
| Codes\\Affect, Embodiment and Identity Themes\Family | 12 |
| Codes\\Affect, Embodiment and Identity Themes\Oppression | 11 |
| Codes\\Affect, Embodiment and Identity Themes\Self-Hate | 9 |
| Codes\\Affect, Embodiment and Identity Themes\Beauty Standards | 8 |
| Codes\\Affect, Embodiment and Identity Themes\Family\Father | 8 |
| Codes\\Health\Mental Health Disorders | 8 |
| Codes\\Affect, Embodiment and Identity Themes\Social Media | 7 |
| Codes\\Affect, Embodiment and Identity Themes\Society | 7 |
| Codes\\Affect, Embodiment and Identity Themes\Representation | 6 |
| Codes\\Affect, Embodiment and Identity Themes\Jealousy or Comparing | 5 |
| Codes\\Affect, Embodiment and Identity Themes\Resistance | 5 |
| Codes\\Feminist New Materialist Theory\Researcher Implication | 5 |
| Codes\\Feminist New Materialist Theory\Speculative Fabulation | 5 |
| Codes\\Affect, Embodiment and Identity Themes\Triggers | 4 |
| Codes\\Affect, Embodiment and Identity Themes\Family\Brother | 3 |
| Codes\\Affect, Embodiment and Identity Themes\Media Influence | 3 |
| Codes\\Affect, Embodiment and Identity Themes\Privilege | 2 |
| Codes\\Feminist New Materialist Theory\Intra-action | 2 |
| Codes\\Feminist New Materialist Theory\Situated Feminisms | 1 |

would be coded under the Sister code. When reviewing the data, as the researcher, I would be able to see that text excerpt coded within both Family and Sister. Feminist New Materialist Theory was included as a parent code to ensure that in the process of analysis I was paying particular attention to my theoretical framework. This parent code includes child codes such as Matter, Situated Feminisms and Intra-Action. Coding within this framework brings to the forefront questions regarding how the research centres materiality and more-than-humans in its affect.

The next parent code, Health, includes three child codes: Healthcare System, Symptoms and Mental Health Disorders. Not included in Table 5.1 are the remainder of codes used in the analysis of the data. The remaining codes were excluded from the presentation of the data in Tables 5.2 and 5.3 because they include identity markers of participants, related parent codes housing child codes that label files with the appropriate participant ID, as well as the participant's identity markers outlined in their screening questionnaire (excluding any true identifying information such as names or specific locations). These parent codes were important during the analysis, as they allowed me to, for example, identify a Twine narrative discussing the effects of healthcare costs and lack of insurance not only by the participant's ID but also by their residence in the United States. This offered me more nuance in analyzing this particular *Click Me* author's experience in a for-profit healthcare system. Finally, Table 5.2 shows the parent code Twine that houses child codes relating to the technological choices and software experiences of the authors and the code frequency. In this parent code, I was able to mark stylistic code choices, narrative path structures, and hyperlink classifications.

## The Abnormal Body

The third most frequently coded theme in the *Click Me* Twine narratives was the topic of the body. This was an expected outcome. The writing prompt offered to authors for constructing their illness narratives asked how it felt to live in a body with hyperandrogenism. The wording of this prompt expectantly produced a body-related narrative from all of the *Click Me* authors. However, it was surprising that every narrative constructed a similar discursive object: the abnormal body. Every *Click Me* author wrote a narrative that framed their body, in some capacity, as an abnormal object. This discursive framing of the abnormal body typically fell into six thematic categories: the abnormal body as uncontrollable, the intense physical and mental labour of maintaining normative femininity, the first menstruation as the initial moment of "discovering" the abnormality of the body, dualized abnormality both in the body and mind, and the abnormal body as a mystery that must be deciphered.

All ten authors employed similar language describing the abnormal body as uncontrollable. Authors constructed the theme of the uncontrollable body by framing the body as requiring control, being uncomfortable, or failing to fit into standard femininity. This concept of the abnormal, uncontrolled body harkens back to Julia Kristeva's concept of the abject, expanded on by scholars such as Judith Butler and detailed in Chapter 2 of this book. Butler argues that there is an exclusionary system at play that produces

*Table 5.2* Twine Code Frequency

| *Code* | *Number of Coding References* |
|---|---|
| Codes\\Twine\Code\Hyperlinks | 176 |
| Codes\\Twine\Twine Structure\Navigational Linking | 111 |
| Codes\\Twine\Twine Structure\Unified Construction | 99 |
| Codes\\Twine\Twine Writing Experience | 69 |
| Codes\\Twine\Code\Style Codes | 65 |
| Codes\\Twine\Twine Structure\Bifold Construction | 38 |
| Codes\\Twine\Twine Software Experiences | 32 |
| Codes\\Twine\Twine Structure\Dead End Linking | 32 |
| Codes\\Twine\Twine Structure\Other Linking | 30 |
| Codes\\Twine\Twine Visuals | 26 |
| Codes\\Twine\Twine Structure\Procedural Linking | 23 |
| Codes\\Twine\Definitions | 9 |
| Codes\\Twine\Twine Structure\Weaving Path | 9 |
| Codes\\Twine\Twine Structure\Multiple Paths | 7 |
| Codes\\Twine\Code\External Links | 5 |
| Codes\\Twine\Twine Structure\Bi-Uni Construction | 5 |
| Codes\\Twine\Twine Structure\Forward Path | 4 |
| Codes\\Twine\Twine Structure\Conversational Linking | 2 |

subjects at the same time that it forms a domain of abject beings, or the not-yet subjects. Butler defined the abject space as "those 'unlivable' and 'uninhabitable' zones of social life which are nevertheless densely populated by those who do not enjoy the status of the subject" (*Bodies That Matter* 3). This concept of the abject situates an idea of excess matter that is seeping out of its proper boundaries. This excess matter is repulsive, useless waste. This concept of the abject body in relation to excess matter is explicit in the narratives of this study. Authors frame their bodily symptoms of hyperandrogenism as abject, excess matter that must be eradicated. There is rarely mention of a lack of bodily matter in association with the disease (hair loss, perhaps, but this symptom was not mentioned frequently). Instead, authors write about unruly, unrelenting dark hair growing on the face like a weed.

They lament the "extra" matter of body fat and "weight" that must be removed from the body. Authors even describe a surplus of menstrual blood flowing from the body. These bodily symptoms are framed, in the narratives, as the excess matter of the unlivable zone and once the matter is overpowered, the body returns to a space of normalcy.

*Click Me* Author 1, for example, writes in their Twine: "I think in a lot of ways living in a body with PCOS is like living in most bodies. Confusing and at times uncontrollable and uncomfortable, but also wonderful." There was a strong thread throughout many narratives of a desire, or requirement, to control the *sick* body. Author 10 writes: "I was convinced that my PCOS was caused by something external and that if I could somehow cut out the 'bad' foods, I'd be cured." Many authors discussed expansive avenues of healing taken throughout their lives, most with the intention to rid their bodies of symptoms. As Author 3 notes: "By stripping myself of my more 'unique' traits, I could finally be [[the fairest of them all]]," they continue that they "Have to remove the abnormality to find the beauty." The abnormal body as a discursive object, for many of the *Click Me* narratives, is framed as a project that requires work, labour, and maintenance in order to restore a state of normality.

In some narratives, the construction of the abnormal body was done in an explicit way. In their story, Author 11 includes a passage with distinct, contrasting lists. The first list appears to include language that describes a normative understanding of womanhood including "no excess hair" and "Menstrates [sic] monthly." Below this list is a second list titled with a hypertext reading "Me." This list includes opposing language to normative femininity such as "Given up on the excess hair battle," and "No menstruation." In other narratives, as reflected in Figure 5.1, this framing of bodily abnormality is done in more abstract ways, including in poetry. The opening passage of Author 5's story, for example, is a poem entitled "Tenebrosity" referring to a state of being dark or shadowed. Author 5 notes in a subsequent passage that "This is how I feel on some days. I feel like staying inside all day, in the dark, never wanting to see the light again." In both of these examples, Authors 11 and 5 paint a picture of shame where one feels cast aside in their difference.

Figure 5.2 depicts a passage from Author 7's Twine story where they describe their experience learning about and coming to terms with their illness diagnosis. Author 7, in this passage, refers to themselves as a "typical case" of hyperandrogenism due to their predictable symptoms. This is a significant language choice because it reveals one of the two ways the *Click Me* authors understand and talk about the abnormal body. In the first way, authors, like Author 7, speak about themselves as the abnormal body. There is no separation between the self and the illness and, in this sense, their body and identity are one. We see this in the way Author 7 declares that they are a

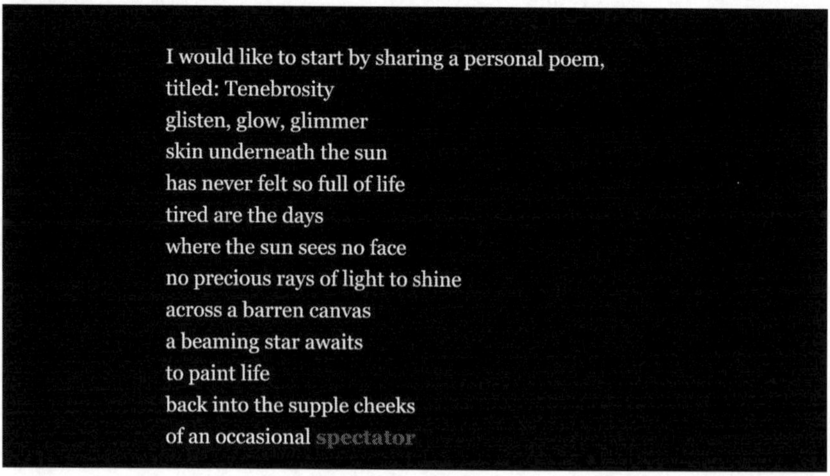

I would like to start by sharing a personal poem,
titled: Tenebrosity
glisten, glow, glimmer
skin underneath the sun
has never felt so full of life
tired are the days
where the sun sees no face
no precious rays of light to shine
across a barren canvas
a beaming star awaits
to paint life
back into the supple cheeks
of an occasional spectator

*Figure 5.1* Screenshot of Author 5's Twine Story.

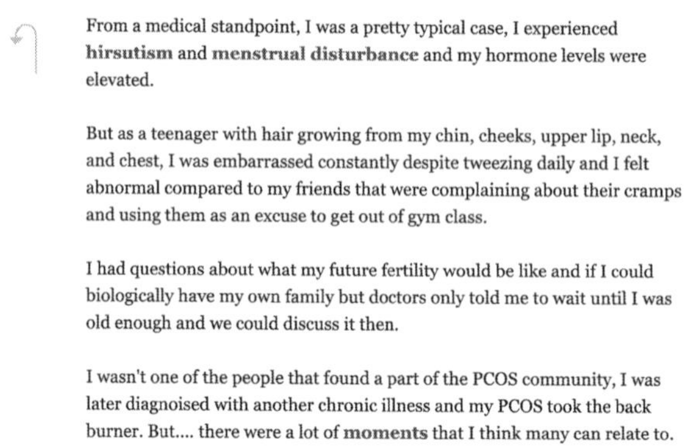

From a medical standpoint, I was a pretty typical case, I experienced **hirsutism** and **menstrual disturbance** and my hormone levels were elevated.

But as a teenager with hair growing from my chin, cheeks, upper lip, neck, and chest, I was embarrassed constantly despite tweezing daily and I felt abnormal compared to my friends that were complaining about their cramps and using them as an excuse to get out of gym class.

I had questions about what my future fertility would be like and if I could biologically have my own family but doctors only told me to wait until I was old enough and we could discuss it then.

I wasn't one of the people that found a part of the PCOS community, I was later diagnoised with another chronic illness and my PCOS took the back burner. But.... there were a lot of **moments** that I think many can relate to.

*Figure 5.2* Screenshot of Author 7's Twine Story.

"typical case" rather than they are experiencing typical symptoms of the illness. This positions the illness as the identity, rather than an external force that has attached to their standard femininity and altered it. In Figure 5.2, Author 7 goes on to ponder what their fertility might be like in the future, not what the disease would do to their "intact by default" fertility. In comparison, a passage in Author 16's story discusses their hopes for their body in the future. In this example, Author 16 uses strong, externalizing language when referring to their body and body parts. They hope that next month "the" skin will become lighter, rather than "their" skin. Author 16 goes on to note: "Maybe my body will love me back the way I want to love it." The author, in this example, refers to their body as an external entity that holds agency and notions of free will separate from themselves. These are important language decisions because Author 16 is framing illness in an opposing way to Author 7 where the body becomes a suit of abnormal skin in which their true self is trapped inside. This creates a distinction between Author 7 who frames illness as something that changes the core of who they are. *Click Me* authors utilized one of these two framing styles, and at times, even oscillated between the two within the same story.

A recurring theme when discussing the abnormal body in author narratives was conveying a sense of intense physical labour to "combat" abnormality or "maintain" normative femininity. In these narratives, the abnormal body is framed as inherently "feminine" where the illness of hyperandrogenism continuously pulls the body into masculinity through unruly symptoms. Through this framing, authors discussed feelings of responsibility to engage in relentless labour practices to "restore" the body to the original state of normality. For example, Author 10 writes: "I met with acupuncturists and therapists. I tried regular massages, starving myself, yoga, countless dietary adjustments and running. [[I tried pleading with my body to get better]]. Nothing worked." One of the most prominent labour practices discussed by authors was body hair removal. Author 1 writes about attending over twenty laser hair removal treatments for facial hair, with no results. The author explains: "For almost a decade now I have been shaving my chin every other day in the shower, hoping that no one ever notices the longer hairs on my chin on the second day." Author 7 describes as a teenager tweezing daily black hairs growing from their chin, cheeks, upper lip, neck and chest. They note that

> There's moments of trying to hide [[hirsutism]], feeling a stray hair outside of the house caused me great anxiety so I began carrying tweezers everywhere I went. Logically I knew the hairs were small but they felt as visible a neon [sic] hazard sign.

This is a compelling passage because the visual of body hair symbolizing a neon hazard sign leads me to wonder what danger it intends to warn against. What kinds of belief systems are functioning that translate human body hair as a public hazard? I read this passage to mean that the author fears their body hair will signal to others that they are ill and/or abnormal and, as a consequence, the author may face social prejudice. This is aligned with Butler's claim that in the process of the body being read as abnormal, the individual moves out of the space of subjecthood as they inhabit the uninhabitable site of abjection (*Bodies that Matter* 3).

Author 3 evokes this process of unrelenting labour related to hair removal in an interesting way. The author uses hypertexts to link back to a previous passage in order to construct a circuit or loop within their Twine narrative. The narrative asks, "what method would you like?" followed by the hypertext options of waxing or threading. If the reader/player chooses to wax, for example, they are brought to a passage that reads:

> The hot wax feels like it burns as its spread thin across my face. Without warning, it is soon ripped off, occassionally [sic] taking bits of the top layer of skin with it due to carelessness. The sensitive skin on my face is left painfully red for the next 24 hours.

Beneath this text is a hypertext that reads "at last, the hair is gone." When the reader/player chooses this hypertext, they are brought to a passage with large black letters that seem to sneer "Just kidding." Below this title the narrative continues: "A week later, the hair sprouts back like a stubborn weed. If I truly want to be [[beautiful]] then this cycle must continue every few weeks. Seemingly endless removal and regrowth." The sole hypertext [[beautiful]] must be chosen to move the narrative to the next passage, however, when the reader/player selects this link, they are looped back to the original passage describing the hair removal methods. This narrative loop designed by the author effectively creates a sense of a loss of agency and an obligation to engage in these labour practices indefinitely. Narrative loops will be discussed in further detail in a later section of this chapter.

Although the *Click Me* Twine narratives repeat some similar experiences of illness, many of the narratives discussed the same initial moment of recognizing the body as abnormal: the first menstruation. This prevalent anecdote found in many of the *Click Me* narratives discusses how the first experience of menstruation deviated from the author's beliefs around "normal" menstruation, including frequency, duration and heaviness. Ultimately, this dissonance between expectations and reality leads the author to understand their bodies as abnormal. Author 4 writes: "My first period started a [[chain reaction]] in my body that would persist for almost two decades." In this narrative, the first menstruation becomes a defining moment in their illness experience and is situated as instigating a domino effect of subsequent symptoms over the course of their life. Author 7 writes: "Like most females, I entered puberty, began developing breasts, body hair, and got my first period. Initally, [sic] my periods came monthly but after six months they became bi-monthly, then annually." In this passage, the author begins by establishing a description of what they believe defines a puberty experience, followed by a stark framing of their different puberty experiences in relation to "most" females. The author writes: "I wasn't comfortable in my own skin and definitely not comfortable discussing my cycle with my family or doctor." The reader comes to understand that the author feels shame in discussing their perception of dysfunctional bodily processes.

When the *Click Me* authors write about the first menstruation as the moment of discovering their body as irregular, there are both over and undertones of sexualization. Not only do the authors become aware of their abnormality during this time, but they are sexualized in their encounters with the healthcare system. Author 1 explains in their interview that they spent time reflecting on their uncomfortable interactions with their male family doctor at a young age during puberty. The author notes that

> I have no idea why I went to see a fertility specialist like it's weird like, finding out you have PCOS when you're young and like your parents are making a lot of medical decisions for you so I have no idea why I had a fertility specialist when I was 14 but I did.

Not only is the author coming to terms with a new identity of being ill but also they are made to understand, by their doctor and parents, that their body's inherent function is to bear children. In some narratives, like Author 1's, the child is sexualized by adults in ways that do not allow for decision-making or agency for the author. In other narratives, there were themes of childhood sexuality that when claimed by the child, yet incite a concealing response in adults. Figure 5.3 shows an excerpt from Author 12's Twine

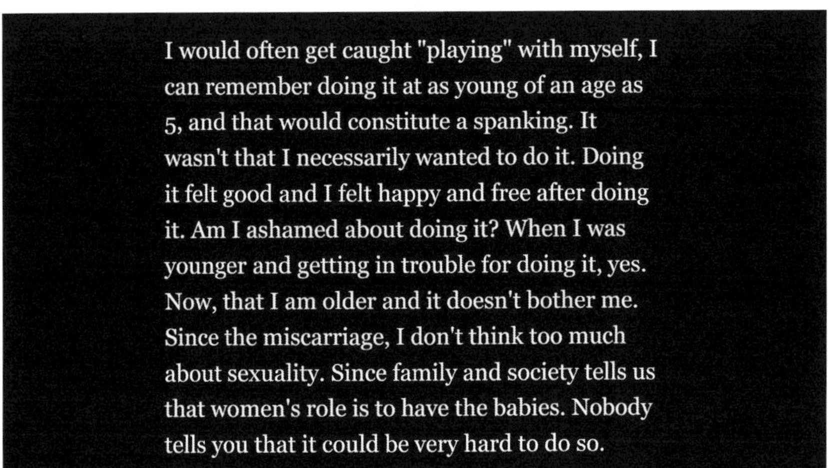
I would often get caught "playing" with myself, I can remember doing it at as young of an age as 5, and that would constitute a spanking. It wasn't that I necessarily wanted to do it. Doing it felt good and I felt happy and free after doing it. Am I ashamed about doing it? When I was younger and getting in trouble for doing it, yes. Now, that I am older and it doesn't bother me. Since the miscarriage, I don't think too much about sexuality. Since family and society tells us that women's role is to have the babies. Nobody tells you that it could be very hard to do so.

*Figure 5.3* Screenshot of Author 12's Twine Story.

story that discusses their memories of experiencing sexual pleasure at a young age, and receiving discipline, including "spanking" from their parents as a result. The author explains that they felt shame from this pleasure in their adolescence because of the response it garnered from the adults around them. However, entering adulthood and experiencing miscarriage has since reshaped their understanding of those earlier experiences. In these two different accounts of childhood sexualization offered by Authors 1 and 12, sexuality is framed as something that can only be imposed onto the body by adults and not discovered or owned by the child themselves.

A strong thread reiterated in the *Click Me* narratives was the concept that the abnormal body is bound to an additional abnormality of emotional issues or nuanced identity. This notion of dualized abnormality, both in identity and body, was constructed in different ways. As described in Chapter 2, I argue in "Illness of the Gendered Body, Freud's *The Uncanny*, and 'Being-in-the-World'" that the phenomenological experience of sex-based illnesses such as hyperandrogenism mirrors the uncanny by rendering the body and therefore identity and selfhood abnormal. A hyperandrogenous body poses the threat of "morphing" into the alien unfamiliar where suddenly one's understanding of their identity in relation to the past and future is challenged. I argue

> With hyperandrogenism, the destabilization of subjecthood is twofold. Supplementing the otherness of our human body, another layer—the gendered body—ties together sociocultural, historical, and political framing of biological sex, bodily appearance, and behaviour. We are not only bodies but gendered bodies.
>
> (Perram, "Illness of the Gendered Body" 594)

When our understanding of health is tied to cultural notions of normative, binary sex expression, a distortion of the body across sexed lines forces one to relinquish their sense of identity. This was mirrored in the *Click Me* narratives in various ways.

Some narratives enforced a perspective that physical abnormality was linked to emotional bankruptcy where the body's sickness is attributed to not being connected to oneself, not doing the "inner" work, and that "healing" is a lifelong journey. In Author 10's narrative, they discuss having a realization that dehumanizing encounters in their life appear to have a correlation to their physical symptoms of bleeding. The author explains that "when my partner would touch me or try to have sex, I would bleed. I noticed that when he would ignore my emotional needs, [[I would bleed]]. I noticed that when I was overworked, I would bleed." In Figure 5.4, Author 10 writes about their experience attending a traditional Indigenous cedar brushing ceremony

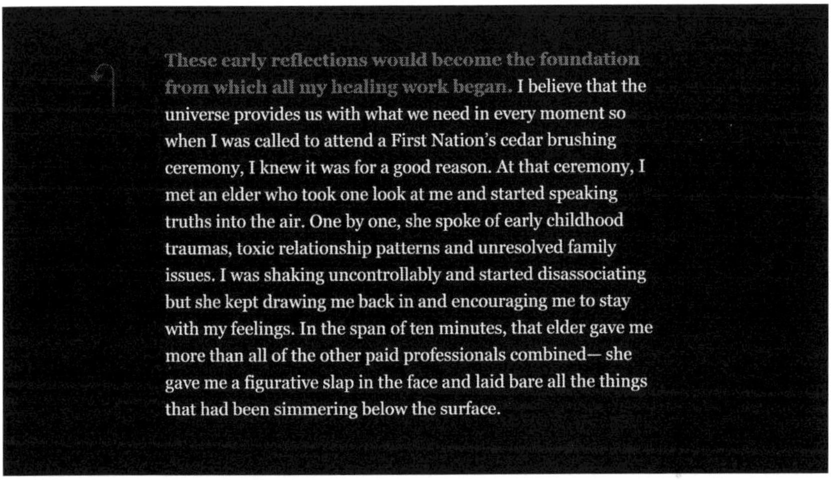
These early reflections would become the foundation from which all my healing work began. I believe that the universe provides us with what we need in every moment so when I was called to attend a First Nation's cedar brushing ceremony, I knew it was for a good reason. At that ceremony, I met an elder who took one look at me and started speaking truths into the air. One by one, she spoke of early childhood traumas, toxic relationship patterns and unresolved family issues. I was shaking uncontrollably and started disassociating but she kept drawing me back in and encouraging me to stay with my feelings. In the span of ten minutes, that elder gave me more than all of the other paid professionals combined– she gave me a figurative slap in the face and laid bare all the things that had been simmering below the surface.

*Figure 5.4* Screenshot of Author 10's Twine Story.

where the advice of an Elder helped forge a new emotional journey for the author. The narrative continues by detailing a series of "self-discovery" endeavours undertaken by the author including ending a harmful relationship, leaving a negative work environment, and establishing boundaries with family members. Author 10 writes: "You may think that PCOS is simply a medical issue but for me, it was rooted in this journey of healing and self-discovery. [[As I began to live in my truth, my symptoms started to ease.]]" For Author 10, the abnormality of the body, in relation to symptoms of hyperandrogenism, is a manifestation of emotional trauma.

Other narratives positioned the concept of the abnormal body as linked to the Queerness of identity. A passage from Author 7's narrative discusses their experiences coming to understand their illness in relation to their Queer identity. They write: "I experienced countless moments of [[embarrassment, feeling abnormal,]] and [[fear of my future]] living with PCOS," they continue:

> For the most part it all became my new 'normal' until I began to question my [[gender]]. The author writes in a subsequent passage that "It took me until 2 to know my favourite colour, until 4 to discover my passion for reading, until 14 to realize I was queer, and until 27 to realize I was non-binary.

In their interview, Author 7 grapples with the question of how intertwined their illness and their gender identity may be. The author considers the relationship between hormonal levels, medication and Queer identity by questioning: "had my hormones not been, like artificially balanced, what would my like sense of being be?" They note a sense of uncertainty with how biological nuances and interventions have come to impact their gender, "because you can't go back and undo it, and then see how somebody's life is gonna turn out." Author 7 notes that they recognize that identifying the relationship between biology and identity is a complex, abstract, inconclusive and possibly dangerous task, however, living with an illness like hyperandrogenism as a nonbinary individual positions you on the frontlines of this debate. The author concludes these thoughts with an insightful description of intersectionality, noting that their illness is one piece of their identity that intersects with the other factors of who they are, including their gender identity and other chronic illnesses.

A final, dominant theme that weaved throughout most of the *Click Me* Twine narratives was the abnormal body as a mystery that requires deciphering. Table 5.1 shows that this theme was coded 32 times as Unknown or Seeking Answers. Many authors wrote passages that discussed, in diverse ways, a deep obligation to uncover the "true" cause of the illness, ultimately to achieve a cure. Author 12, for example, writes that their mother was asked to bring the author back to the hospital for further testing after their birth, but the results came back missing or inconclusive. The author laments:

> I am not sure if a blood test would be something that could really prove that a baby has all the markers that would could [sic] predict that they might have PCOS in the future. That would be an interesting thing to study.

The author suggests that identifying the illness early in life would have value for those affected. We see this similar quest for answers in Author 7's story. The author discusses receiving a report of ovarian cysts that validated their PCOS diagnosis and "also an increased sense of uncertainty. How long have I had cysts? When did they develop? Are they stable or growing?" Answering one question, for this author, mushrooms into a series of further questions that require answers. Author 3 writes about their journey in seeking an answer to what was causing their symptoms. In Figure 5.5, Author 3 describes feelings of relief upon receiving an official PCOS diagnosis. The author explains that the desire to search for answers and the "root" of the illness stems from a need to relieve themselves of a sense of guilt that they may have "caused" their bodily symptoms. PCOS, in this sense, becomes an external force that enacts deviance onto the author, and with the illness label, the author is relinquished of responsibility for their abnormal body.

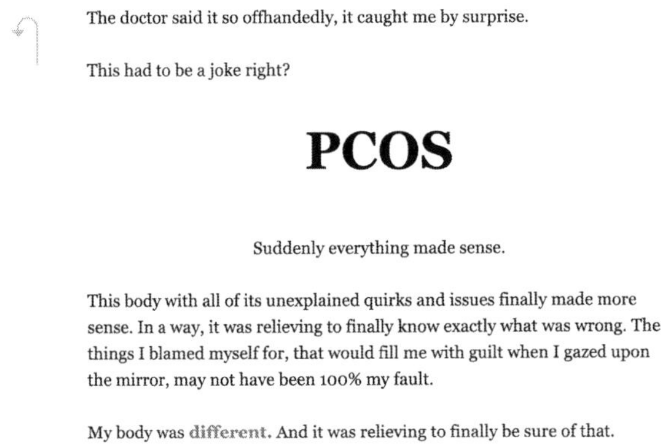

The doctor said it so offhandedly, it caught me by surprise.

This had to be a joke right?

**PCOS**

Suddenly everything made sense.

This body with all of its unexplained quirks and issues finally made more sense. In a way, it was relieving to finally know exactly what was wrong. The things I blamed myself for, that would fill me with guilt when I gazed upon the mirror, may not have been 100% my fault.

My body was different. And it was relieving to finally be sure of that.

*Figure 5.5* Screenshot B of Author 3's Twine Story.

## Narratives of Relationality

All the *Click Me* narratives include compelling and nuanced accounts of the ways in which relationships with other people come to form meaning around the illness experience. In this section, relationality, as an affective force that generates kinship and connection, will be discussed as an agent of relationships in the narrative story. The *Click Me* authors show in their narratives that the ways in which they come to understand themselves as *sick* are formed not solely by the experience of symptoms, but through their encounters with other people. The most prevalent relationships coded in the narratives include the relationship with the mother, the sister and the romantic partner. Themes that emerged around the mother include shame in revealing the abnormality of the body to the mother, the mother's role to gatekeep the normality of the daughter's body, fear of becoming your mother and fear of not experiencing motherhood. Narratives that included the theme of the sister centred on jealousy, comparison and a belief structure that the sister is outperforming womanhood. Finally, themes around the romantic partner include anxieties around illness disrupting the body's sexual appeal and actions of a supportive versus an unsupportive partner.

The narratives in this study were saturated with themes of the mother. Table 5.1 shows that the concept of the Mother was coded twenty-eight times and more than any other family member. It became evident, in the analysis of the narratives, that the idea of the mother and conceptualizations of motherhood are foundational belief systems that construct the way authors have come to understand hyperandrogenism and their bodies. A typical initial mention of the mother in the narratives correlated to the first menstruation anecdotes discussed in a previous section of this chapter. When the author first perceives that their menstruation is abnormal, there is collective anxiety in having to reveal this to the mother. Author 1 writes:

> My first period lasted for 6 months. I was too emberassed [sic] to talk to my mother about my period, and none of my friend [sic] had theirs at the time, so I continued to navigate dramatically irregular periods for a few years, before I got up the courage to talk to my mom about it.

In the authors' narratives, there is a common thread of shame around revealing to the mother that the body was not, in fact, "progressing" into womanhood as expected. Author 11 writes: "Summoning the courage as a 16 year old girl to tell your mom you've missed your last couple [[periods->Opening Passage]]." For Author 11, disclosing to the mother their lack of menstruation is an act that requires courage. This shame and fear described by authors appears to come to a crux at a collective perception that the mother desires normative femininity for the daughter. We see this in a passage from Author 3's narrative where they describe their belief that their mother only finds them beautiful when they successfully "rid" the body of their masculinizing traits such as excess facial hair.

Going deeper into the belief structure that the mother desires normative femininity for the daughter revealed that it was not just a desire but also the mother's role to maintain the daughter's normalcy. Through various narrative anecdotes, coloured by the ways in which authors constructed meaning, there is a notion that the mother's job is to monitor the normality of the daughter's body and to intervene when dysfunction is perceived. Author 1 constructs this belief system effectively in their narrative. The author writes about their mother first taking them to visit the doctor to address their absent periods as a teenager, but soon they would attend appointments on their own to assert their "independence as a young woman." Following receiving a diagnosis of PCOS and discussions of future infertility, Author 1 writes:

> This stuck with me because when I returned home my mother asked me about my appointment and I distinctly remember her being very upset about this one piece of information. Up until I told my mother I had not been that concerned about possible infertility. But my mother's reaction made me wonder if I should be more concerned.

In Figure 5.6, Author 1 explains that their mother, throughout their life, focused excessively on the daughter's potential infertility. Before the author's wedding, the mother told the author that they should disclose their potential infertility to their future mother-in-law. The author writes: "I felt a bit like a

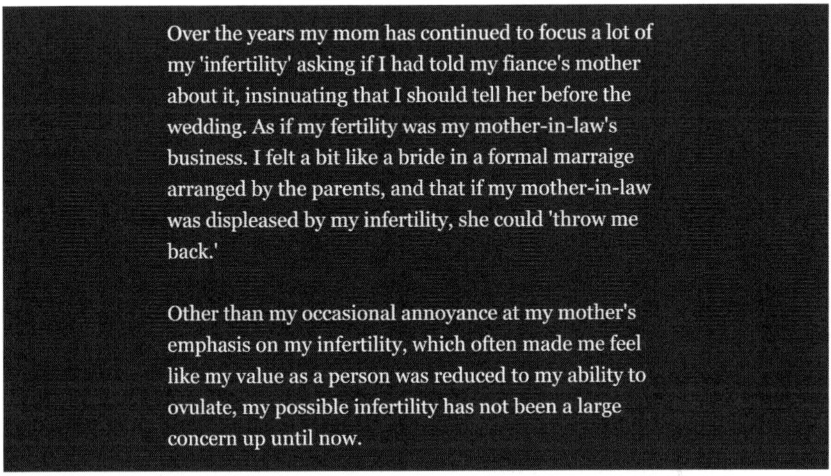

Over the years my mom has continued to focus a lot of my 'infertility' asking if I had told my fiance's mother about it, insinuating that I should tell her before the wedding. As if my fertility was my mother-in-law's business. I felt a bit like a bride in a formal marraige arranged by the parents, and that if my mother-in-law was displeased by my infertility, she could 'throw me back.'

Other than my occasional annoyance at my mother's emphasis on my infertility, which often made me feel like my value as a person was reduced to my ability to ovulate, my possible infertility has not been a large concern up until now.

*Figure 5.6* Screenshot A of Author 1's Twine Story.

bride in a formal marrige [sic] arranged by the parents, and that if my mother-in-law was displeased by my infertility, she could 'throw me back.'" Through the ways in which Author 1 writes about their experiences with infertility in relation to their mother, the author becomes objectified. In this formation, the author is reduced to an object of ovulation, and the mother becomes the agent of femininity maintenance.

An anchoring theme at the centre of relationality was both implicit and explicit fear of becoming the mother. Becoming the mother figure, for authors, was both physical in terms of "inheriting" an illness or experiencing masculinizing symptoms, and emotions relating to the mother's disposition and her beliefs about the world. This theme was most strongly constructed in Author 12's narrative in compelling ways. The initial mention of the mother in this narrative begins when the author is describing their first months of pregnancy:

> The congratulations start and I am reminded of what my mom told me in the past about her having at least one miscarriage. This isn't my mom's story, I think to myself. It's mine, and it will have a better outcome.

Author 12 goes on to describe a cruel and complicated mother. A child of the 1960s, with "progressive" views on women's liberation, she was often combative with the author's father who was a dangerous man, suspicious of doctors and the education system. In one passage, the author describes how their mother and aunt would take them shopping in the boy's section. The author writes: "She and my aunt would often tease me about my body, the clothes I wear, and asking me what I would do with a husband. While I was a teenager, I had no idea." In another passage, Author 12 describes watching their mother lament plucking "disgusting, long, black hairs" from her face, then "she would tell me to come closer and would proceed to pluck the hairs off my face as well." The author's declaration that "this isn't my mom's story" is a compelling, generative statement. What is generated is, in fact, a version of the mother's story told by the experiences of the daughter. It is a narrative about a struggle to sever self-identity from the mother, but in this pursuit, the mother's story becomes deeply intertwined with the daughter's.

A strong but inverse theme of fear around becoming the mother was fear around not becoming a mother at all. This topic was expected to emerge in the narratives. Infertility is a common symptom of PCOS, and concerns about the ability to conceive were a theme in the *Click Me* screening interviews. However, the way in which infertility was written about in the narratives was specific. Issues around current infertility were mentioned, however, most authors spoke about the diagnosis of PCOS igniting a life-long fear of the future regarding motherhood. In many narratives, after receiving a PCOS diagnosis as a teenager, no further medical intervention is taken but the author is told to visit the doctor when they want to get pregnant. This fertility anticipation creates a looming sense of uncertainty for the author's future and, at times, positions them to contemplate their intentions for parenthood before their peers. Author 7 writes:

> Initally, [sic] I felt extremely disconnected from my diagnosis, I wasn't necessarily 'unwell', my body was just functioning differently. The root of my fear was thinking about my future. I had always wanted to be a parent and PCOS seemed to be stealing this way from me.

For this author, they had constructed an idea of their future, and a diagnosis of PCOS disrupts this trajectory. Author 9's narrative centres on the experience of trying to become pregnant. In one passage, the author describes receiving their first vaginal ultrasound where they were not "prepared at how invasive it was, but I pretended not to care." Through the outcomes of this test, the author learns that there is a strong chance they will experience infertility, as they note: "And that was the beginning. The beginning of a life-long struggle." For Authors 7 and 9 a life path of anxiety around the potential of motherhood emerges alongside the illness diagnosis.

In reflecting on the larger veins of meaning that flow from the analysis of the mother it would be simple to conclude that the mother, in the narratives of this study, is a domineering presence that is generally harmful to the positive identity formative for the author. However, when we dig deeper into this construction of the mother, concepts of internalized misogyny emerge. In light of the negative portrayals of the mother characters in these narratives,

I wonder if there is space to consider the social roles we place on motherhood and how we frame failure as a society, in this context. After all, mothers, in many cases, stand as primary caregivers, both physically and emotionally for children. Factors that could be considered here include what support mothers receive, possible misattribution of the mother's impact, roles of other parents, and societal judgement of the mother's behaviour. In their interview, Author 1 astutely reflects on the way in which writing about the negative experiences of illness led to narratively constructing their mother in a similar light. They note: "And so at the beginning, I was writing like really negative things about like my experiences with doctors and the way that my mom had reacted, especially, which was weird. I was like, 'oh, why am I like villainizing my mom?'" The author goes on to note: "She's, like, probably my most like, formative person." This encapsulates, in this research, how relationality comes to shape narrative construction. The mother, like the illness, becomes a dominant oppressor. They become intertwined and interchangeable.

The second most prevalent family member to be referenced in the narratives of the *Click Me* authors was the sister. Reference to the sister was made 14 times throughout author stories, and the majority of these references unearthed themes of resentment in being compared to the sister, particularly because of a perception that the sister is performing womanhood more effectively than the author. Author 11 discusses in a passage the moment when their sister happily reveals two positive pregnancy tests. Emotionally exhausted from their own infertility journey, the author reflects on responding with jealousy and ultimately ruining their sister's joyful moment. Later, in our closing interview, Author 11 revisited this moment in their narrative and concluded that participating in this study and writing about their illness experience helped re-contextualize their response to their sister's pregnancy news. They explain:

> there was the part in there where I talked about, like my sister getting pregnant. That was a really big moment, because she actually just found out she's pregnant again. We reacted much differently this time…but I'm realizing that it was the shame that was actually causing that, like, the fact that I've been working so hard and couldn't get something that's so easy for other people. I think it gave me a better understanding of the emotions attached to it, I guess.

A similar sentiment emerges in the narrative of Author 12. This author discusses how their sister was always deemed "the beautiful one" who received endless gifts from men who were interested in her. The author explains that rather than feeling emotions of jealousy, they noticed a stark difference in how the world treated them. The author writes: "There was a difference."

Their mother, for example, would ask the author why they could not be more like their sister. What reference to the sister in these narratives reveals is, rather than a literal sibling, the sister becomes a symbolic concept of a feminine ideal that the illness of hyperandrogenism prevents the author from achieving.

A final, albeit significant, relationship code was that of romantic partners. This theme was coded 28 times throughout author narratives under the Relationship code. Discussions of romantic relationships in the Twine narratives were diverse but relatively fell into one of three themes. First, authors discussed feeling as if the disease of hyperandrogenism strips them of femininity and therefore renders them undesirable to romantic partners. Second, in longer-term heterosexual relationships, authors wrote about feeling as if they are failing in their role of womanhood, a role that is required of them in a romantic partnership. Finally, there was ample discussion of moments of unsupportive actions from a romantic partner in contrast to the partner acting as the sole, safe companion to discuss anxieties and fears regarding the illness.

Author 1 includes a passage in their narrative dedicated to their experiences of not feeling desirable to men because of their hyperandrogenism symptoms. The hypertext that grants access to this passage is labelled, in the narrative, as [[Dating: a Hairy Situation]]. Figure 5.7 details the author's experience dating with excess body hair. They describe how body hair, particularly on their chin, made them insecure as they feared a partner would touch their face and feel the pricks of stubble. They note that it took time to share their vulnerabilities with their current husband, and enough trust has built between them that the author often shaves their face in front of him.

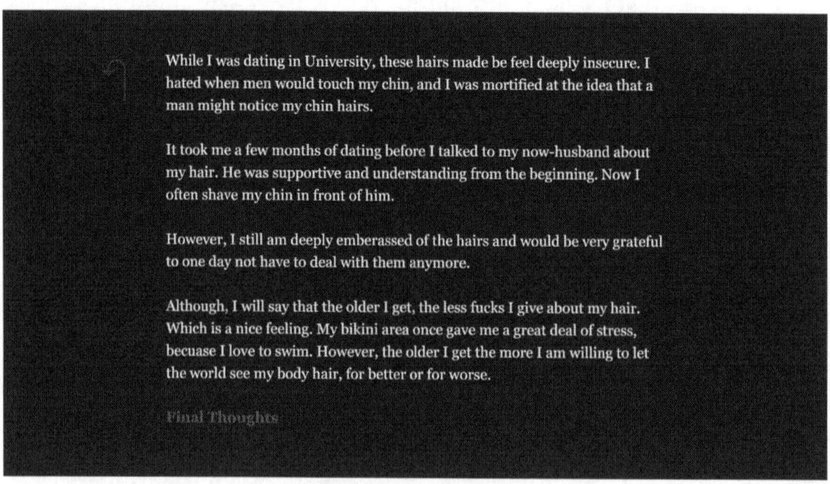
While I was dating in University, these hairs made be feel deeply insecure. I hated when men would touch my chin, and I was mortified at the idea that a man might notice my chin hairs.

It took me a few months of dating before I talked to my now-husband about my hair. He was supportive and understanding from the beginning. Now I often shave my chin in front of him.

However, I still am deeply emberassed of the hairs and would be very grateful to one day not have to deal with them anymore.

Although, I will say that the older I get, the less fucks I give about my hair. Which is a nice feeling. My bikini area once gave me a great deal of stress, becuase I love to swim. However, the older I get the more I am willing to let the world see my body hair, for better or for worse.

Final Thoughts

*Figure 5.7* Screenshot B of Author 1's Twine Story.

The author concludes this passage by explaining how time has helped them to gain more confidence in their body. Where they once used to feel ashamed of the hair on their inner thighs when they would wear a bathing suit, they now swim in public with body hair exposed.

Author 11 discusses feelings around perceived blame in their partnership, particularly in relation to the author's perceptions around their body failing to perform womanhood as expected. The author discusses their long and painful journey with infertility in their marriage:

> I know the suffering is not just my own. My spouse, excited as he was at the first positive also feels the pain of each negative test as well. Sometimes I think he blames me. And I don't fault him on that. I blame [[me->Opening Passage]] too.

This passage is compelling and speaks to underlying assumptions around gender roles in heterosexual relationships as well as assumptions around health and illness. There are belief systems emerging that establish the female body as inherently fertile and when a heterosexual couple is unable to get pregnant there is an assumption that it is a failure of the female body. This removes the role of the male body in fertility while also establishing binaries of biological sex and health: healthy women are always fertile and therefore not conceiving means the women's body is *sick*.

Finally, author narratives conveyed vivid anecdotes that explored what support looks like to the author in a partnership. For example, Author 9 explained that their husband acted as their support system because: "he comforts me when I feel physical pain brought upon by my medications, and emotional pain brought about my period [sic] (aka when my medications did not work)." This is in contrast to Author 10 who writes about what an unsupportive partnership looks like to them. They describe attending a couples therapy session with their partner of a decade where the therapist asks to see the author alone for the next session. In this private meeting, the therapist advises the author to end the relationship with their partner. The author notes how difficult it was to come to terms with this advice, but ultimately it helped them begin to make other large changes in various aspects of their life. The romantic partner, in many of the author narratives, stands as a robust, dynamic symbol: the partner may be a stable, safe force, a site of instability, or a space to project fear of rejection.

## Healthcare Experience

Table 5.1 shows that the second most frequently coded theme was Healthcare System Experiences. Narrative reference to healthcare, in any way, was made 95 times in author narratives. Although the *Click Me* module's writing prompt centred the embodied experience of the disease, grappling with experiences in the healthcare system was a recurring topic throughout author screening and closing interviews, as well. Similarly, in the political framing section of the Twine module, there are passages that reference the experience of visiting the doctor with hyperandrogenism. The module calls the reader to consider: "Anxious? Alone? Optimistic? Cared for? Dismissed? How do you feel when you visit the doctor?" The following passage reads: "Some women* with hyperandrogenism have had negative experiences at the doctor's office. They feel: They weren't listened to. Their symptoms were dismissed. They weren't treated like a person." The subsequent passages situate the disease as a collective experience by describing how, despite a lack of awareness, hyperandrogenism is a prevalent condition that many individuals live with. The module then leads the author to consider methods, such as creative writing, to respond to the emotional impacts of the disease. It is likely that these passages that frame hyperandrogenism's intersection with the healthcare system led authors to consider their own healthcare experiences and possibility reflect on them in their narratives.

The *Click Me* authors, overwhelmingly, framed their experiences in the healthcare system as negative, mainly through feeling subjugated, dehumanized, or dismissed by their physicians. An additional negative experience included perceiving the physician to lack knowledge on the topic of PCOS. Figure 5.8 shows a passage from Author 10's story where the author describes feeling their symptoms are dismissed by their physician despite experiencing concerning symptoms. The physician, in the narrative, notes that he does not recognize any signs of abnormality, as the author explains: "Once again he

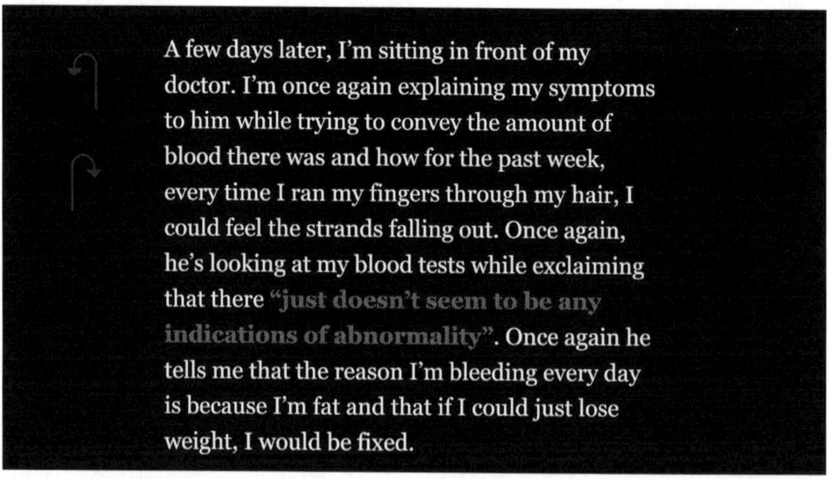


*Figure 5.8* Screenshot of Author 10's Twine Story.

tells me that the reason I'm bleeding every day is because I'm fat and that if I could just lose weight, I would be fixed." The next passage in the author's story is a single line that reads: "I want to spit in his face. But I don't." This anecdote creates a dynamic understanding of what constitutes abnormality for the physician that centres around blame.

The physician, in this story, seems to link the term abnormality, not to unexpected bodily symptoms that distress the patient, but rather, to some sort of core, buried, inherent bodily malfunction. The abnormality, in this case, would not be the "fault" of the patient, but rather something biologically faulty. The author's body size, in contrast, is framed by the physician as both the fault of the patient and the cause of the symptoms. In other words, the physician is putting forward a belief system in which the patient is not classified as abnormal because this designation is reserved for individuals who lack control over their circumstances, and, perhaps, did not cause their condition. For the physician, true abnormality possesses a fundamental deficiency for which they do not hold blame. The physician perceives the patient as engaging in poor moral decisions that lead to weight gain and subsequent health issues. Through this belief system, abnormality is a classification assigned to those without culpability.

Author 10 revisits this narrative moment in our closing interview where they describe viewing TikTok content that explores women's dehumanizing experiences of "being fat at the doctor's office." The author explains that encountering other women who had similar experiences was a validating and community-building moment for them. The author explains: "I would say like writing [the] experience and reflecting on the whole like fatphobic doctor thing that was kind of powerful for me because I was like, it just reaffirms, you know what I've always been thinking," mainly that "there's really a lot of fatphobic doctors out there that just think that fat is like that's the only problem and then if you could just get rid of the fat that everything else would be like fine." Ultimately, the author notes that it was the process of writing about the experience in conjunction with finding kinship with other women that allowed them to feel validation.

A thematic throughline in many author narratives was experiences of violation during particular medical procedures, mainly transvaginal ultrasounds. Author 12 describes receiving their first Papanicolaou test as a young adult and feeling fear because they lacked instructional communication on what to expect. The author describes: "Each time I have a pap done, I feel a little violated, I think due to the invasiveness of the procedure. The doctors were female, and told me they would be gentle." This is a similar sentiment articulated by Author 9 who wrote: "It was my first vaginal ultrasound. I was not prepared at how invasive it was, but **I pretended not to care**." The author's coded emphasis on the phrase "I pretended not to care" centres the idea that the author was compelled to camouflage their feelings of violation during the procedure, rather than intervene. This anecdote raises questions about how patients with hyperandrogenism might come to understand their role in the healthcare encounter and the level of agency or bodily autonomy they hold in that setting.

How relationality comes to shape experience was a recurring theme in both the *Click Me* narratives and the closing interviews where authors reflected on how the entanglements of matter, identities, histories, biology and technology impact negative healthcare outcomes. One interpretation of this theme might be intersectionality, a term that was used by several authors to describe their experience. As explored in Chapter 3, however, this book will frame the phenomenon as assemblage theory. As Jasbir K. Puar argues, "transnational, postcolonial, and critical race theorists have pointed out, the centrality of the subject positioning of white women has been re-secured through the way in which intersectionality has been deployed" (373). Puar calls for a Queer assemblage framework to supplement the short-comings of intersectionality (372). As discussed in Chapter 3, in some ways that intersectionality has been taken up, identity is positioned as a product of a gridlock where individual identities can be teased out and their impact analyzed in isolation. Assemblage theory centres the evolution of the identity, not as a collection of parts, but as an entanglement of relations that cannot be reduced to individualized identities. Assemblage theory accounts for how *things* inside and outside identity are, in fact, that identity as well. Assemblage theory, in this project, is an expansion not a rejection of intersectionality. As Puar argues, the two theories are not oppositional but "frictional" to each other (372). This friction is important for understanding the experience of hyperandrogenism because although feminist new materialism is centred as the theoretical framework of this research, the *Click Me* authors used the term intersectionality to describe their experiences.

In a passage from Author 4's narrative, they discuss the frustration they feel about a perceived lack of equality or fairness for patients in the healthcare system. They go on to write: "There is comfort knowing that we have a community, because talking about PCOS and Hyperandrogenism will eventually normalize it. May this be the start to more dialogue, more assistance, and a better understanding of this condition." In our closing interview, Author 4 expands on this moment by offering a nuancing of their experience. Author 4 explains that as a Person of Colour, it was, in fact, surprising to them that their own experience in the healthcare system was brief and effective. This is because, as the author explains:

> with a bunch of news coming out about People of Colour and, you know, just different minorities being mistreated at the hands of healthcare professionals—it's—I've become acutely aware that I'm probably one of the luckier ones for sure.

Author 4 highlights the ways in which race intersects with illness to further perpetuate a risk of mistreatment in the healthcare system.

Author 7 similarly draws attention to moments of intersectionality when thinking about gender identity in relation to the healthcare system. In our closing interview, Author 7 and I had a lengthy and nuanced conversation about the experience of being nonbinary and having hyperandrogenism. Author 7 touched on insightful and complex factors that have made their illness experience different than a cisgender woman with the same disease. The author reflected on the supremacy of the biomedical model and its perceived inability to make space for diverse gender identities. They explain that, in their experience, PCOS is a "female-dominated condition" where the specialists they have visited are "just looking at your biological parts" and have not been appropriately trained in gender diversity. Author 7 concludes that: "it's a big assumption that if you have this, that you're female, and that's just like the world that it is." Ultimately, the author points to not only a gap in the standard education of physicians but the impacts of larger sociocultural systems that lead to discrimination of gender-diverse people in the healthcare system.

A unique but significant theme detailed by one author was the impacts of capitalism and the healthcare system. Author 12 was an American resident, and their narrative touched on the impacts of healthcare costs and insurance in ways that other authors did not. It was apparent, as confirmed in our closing interview, that Author 12 attended medical facilities that utilize a different healthcare model than other authors in the study, presumably the Canadian universal healthcare system (which has its own critical issues). Author 12, as an American, would be referencing encounters in medical facilities that may be operated by one of the many distinct organizations or private-sector businesses, including non-profit organizations, government, or for-profit companies, that function in their country of residence. Author 12 shares a sobering anecdote about attending the hospital during a miscarriage. Before the author is able to see a physician, and while they are still actively bleeding from the miscarriage, they are directed to pay for the medical services. The author explains:

> We are directed to wait even longer, so that we can talk to someone at finance. I am still bleeding, waiting to see a doctor about a child that could be growing inside of me. They show us into an office where they explain all of the charges. We agree to the terms of paying them anything that we would owe. [[Then we go back to the waiting room]].

Author 12 goes on to describe being wheeled to a private room to receive an abdominal ultrasound where the healthcare provider asks the author if they are interested in receiving a transvaginal ultrasound as well. The author explains:

> I have no idea what it is and they tell me that I could opt out of it if I wanted to. I ask if it's going to cost more and if I would have to do it again in a few days anyhow. The answer to these questions are yes.

The author notes that they decline the procedure, which they and their partner later regret. In our closing interview, Author 12 expands on how they believe their experience with this hospital's approach to receiving payment for services, and how they processed this, was impacted by their profession. The author had worked as a data-analyst for a hospital in the past and described that they were constantly reminded of the organization's priority to make the hospital as much money as possible, despite that fact, as the author explains: "this was a non-for-profit hospital." Although Author 12 was the only author to discuss the impacts of fee structures for medical services, this is a significant, additional barrier that patients with hyperandrogenism may face in differing healthcare systems.

The dominant narrative theme of negative healthcare experiences is framed by the *Click Me* authors in opposition to what they identified as positive experiences, mainly feeling validated, heard and understood by physicians. Author 11 sets up an effectively dizzying hypertext circuit where the reader/player must click through various hypertexts labelled as [[Dr. 1]], [[Dr. 2]], [[Dr. 3]] and [[Dr. 4]]. Selecting [[Dr. 1]] brings the reader/player to a passage that discusses the author visiting a physician with their mother at 16 years old. The physician tells the author to return when they plan to have children, reminiscent of Arthur Frank's concept of "remission society" that calls on the author to return to the healthcare system later, leaving them "well but not cured" (8). Selecting the [[Dr. 2]] hypertext brings the reader/player to a passage that reads: "He had never HEARD of PCOS and seemed like something that was over diagnosed. Refused me any help with it." This sentiment of dismissal is reflected again in the [[Dr. 4]] passage where the author describes how the physician ignored their diagnosis but offered options to remove the patient's "unsightly" skin tags. While the author establishes a sense of perpetual dismissal in their physician encounters, the cycle is broken when the reader/player selects the [[Dr. 3]] hypertext. Here, the author reverses the previous formula by describing a female physician who was akin to "sunshine." The author describes that this physician was empathetic and understanding of their illness and she progressed the author's treatment by making referrals to specialists and facilitating regular blood work and medication refills.

The other *Click Me* authors use similar descriptive language to write about physicians who facilitate positive relationships. Author 10 wrote that their physician "was patient and understood that my past trauma was going to make it difficult to insert the IUD but she was persistent yet gentle when booking me for another appointment to try again." Author 7 refers to their physician as "friendly, validating, and extremely comforting" in expressing to the author that they would address their illness. What is compelling about this thematic dichotomy created by the authors about what constitutes a negative versus a positive patient-physician encounter is that there was a distinct interpretation of gendered dynamics. A sustained belief from authors was that a male physician tended to be present in negative healthcare encounters whereas a female physician may facilitate positive experiences. This belief system was rarely articulated directly by authors, however, it was continually insinuated through various language choices.

When authors chose to include or exclude the gender of the physician it created rich, generative meaning in the narrative context. It became apparent that when a *Click Me* author typically names a character as the "doctor" in their narrative, but suddenly makes a choice to include a sole reference to this same character as the "male doctor" or the "female doctor," there was something intentional happening. The author is making a statement that the gender of the physician becomes important in the way they make meaning from their story. For example, in our closing interview, Author 10 discusses "the other doctor that I found, like the female doctor" and "how she was so much more patient." Author 12 writes in their narrative how "The female doctor arrives and she tells me that the miscarriage was 'complete'. I think she may be crying as she tells me." Although assumptions can be drawn regarding why authors may have established this gendered dynamic, including perhaps a perception that female physicians may have lived experiences with sex-based illness embodiment, the *Click Me* narratives did not expand deep into this territory.

Finally, the *Click Me* authors, in many ways, positioned alternative approaches to their illness in opposition to normative healthcare practices. Author 12 creates this dichotomy in their Twine story by creating two separate hypertext links labelled [[Naturopathic Doctor]] and [[Western Medicine]]. Selecting the latter brings the reader/player through a narrative plot detailing the author's negative, dehumanizing experiences in the normative healthcare system. When the former hypertext is selected, a different story emerges. Here, Author 12 writes a detailed narrative about feeling as if they had no path forward in the normative healthcare system. The author discusses feeling frustrated with being prescribed antibiotics every few months for a chronic condition that would not subside. The author's husband, on a flight back from China, met a flight attendant who suggested his wife see a naturopathic doctor. The author was sceptical about the validity of this practice. Their mother shamed them for considering this option and posed a series of questions to the author including: "What if it's a hoax?" and "Have you lost your mind?"

Author 12 decides to visit a naturopathic doctor, whom they describe as

> wearing busines [sic] casual underneath a lab coat and a stethoscope and does not look nearly as old as she is. Her hair is put up in a graceful way, something about her is different from anyone else I have met and it is a bit scary at first.

The naturopathic doctor engages in consultation with the author and ultimately prescribes them a series of remedies the author has never considered before, including a food intolerance test, a bedtime routine, reflecting on their troubled relationship with their father, thoroughly chewing food, and a seed rotation that involves integrating various seeds in relation to the body's hormonal cycle and the moon cycle. The naturopathic doctor also advises the author to take more time to enjoy life, where the author laments: "No doctors prescribe fun." The author concludes their narrative with a strong endorsement of their experience with naturopathic medicine and discusses how they feel both physically and emotionally better. Ultimately, the author notes that the naturopathic doctor "asked me more questions that any other doctor had in my life. It was really wonderful to work with her as she knows the word 'doctor' means 'teacher'... I trust her with my life." In our closing interview, when reflecting on this narrative moment, Author 12 explained that they are going to continue using naturopathic medicine to address their illness because: "I felt more. I felt loved."

Author 10 creates a similar dichotomy between normative healthcare practices and alternative approaches to illness, which for the author is emotional healing work in relation to mind-body connections. As shown previously in Figure 5.4, this author details a compelling anecdote in their Twine narrative where, at the depth of their illness, they were invited to an Indigenous cedar brushing ceremony where they met an Elder who helped them start to make deep emotional connections. The author explains:

> In the span of ten minutes, that elder gave me more than all of the other paid professionals combined–she gave me a figurative slap in the face and laid bare all the things that had been simmering below the surface.

This experience led the author to begin to reframe their illness and approach it in a different way—as an embodied emotional response to trauma where once the trauma is addressed the physical symptoms will resolve.

There is an intriguing connection between Author 12 and 10's narrative construction of alternative illness response methods. Rather than centring if and how the physical methods alleviate symptoms of the body, it seems that the authors are highlighting the transformative potential of a connected relationality. Where the authors frame normative healthcare encounters as subjecting and dehumanizing, they position alternative approaches as empowering, generative and personally profound. Rather than interrogating if alternative responses to illness "work" in the sense that they produce a measurable reduction of physical symptoms, the authors seem to be highlighting that these practices "work" because they make them feel heard, understood and validated in their illness experience. Author 12 explains their naturopathic doctor "told me that I was not 'broken' there's nothing 'wrong' with me," and this validation that their body was not, in fact, abnormal, seems to be a strong source of the author's support of an alternative approach to illness.

## Empowerment

A common bookend theme in many of the *Click Me* author narratives was that of empowerment. Table 5.1 shows the theme of Empowerment was coded in the author narratives 23 times, directly, however, this theme in various interpretations emerged in other codes as well. Authors discussed the theme of empowerment generally in three specific ways: knowledge and/or receiving a diagnosis, transformation and community-building. The majority of the *Click Me* Twine narratives explored themes of trauma, powerlessness or subjugation, however, there was a common literary strategy to pull the narrative conclusion into a moment of empowered summation. These conclusions focused on outlining strategies, approaches and tactics that have allowed the author to feel more empowered in their illness journey.

A strong, recurring perspective perpetuated through multiple narratives was that acquiring knowledge on hyperandrogenism, or receiving a formal diagnosis of the disease, was an empowering experience for the author. Author 3 describes a moment when their physician informs them of their diagnosis for the first time: "This body with all of its unexplained quirks and issues finally made more sense." The author explains,

> In a way, it was relieving to finally know exactly what was wrong. The things I blamed myself for, that would fill me with guilt when I gazed upon the mirror, may not have been 100% my fault. My body was different. And it was relieving to finally be sure of that.

This embracing of the potential of difference harkens back to Coleman et al.'s analysis of difference as feminist new materialism anti-prejudice energy that is generative rather than inhibiting, discussed in Chapter 3. Coleman et al. explain: "it takes us away from thinking difference only as binary separation or as opposed to sameness. It is entirely new and fresh thinking of difference: it affirms rather than negates." Difference, here, builds up rather than divides as, and according to feminist new materialism, it is not concerned with separatism but multiplicity.

In one passage, Author 3 offers three hypertext options to describe their newfound perception of themselves: [[Understanding]], [[Acceptance]] and

[[Empowerment]]. Selecting the first hypertext brings the reader/player to a lengthy passage describing how a diagnosis helped the author understand themselves and their place in the world, including cultivating a sense of pride in being represented when learning about their illness in university courses. The second hypertext link, [[Acceptance]], explores how the author found acceptance within groups of people like them, and within themselves, including finding kinship in Facebook groups dedicated to the illness and within their own family with family members who also had the disease. Finally, selecting the [[Empowerment]] hyperlink leads the reader/player to a passage in which the author describes feeling newly emboldened to advocate for others marginalized by the disease. The author writes:

> I am now more empowered than ever to use my voice to advocate for others like me. Those that are lost, that are trying to accept themselves, that feel ostracized for the way their bodies look or behave, I can advocate for. I want to build a future where those who are struggling with themselves can live as they wish.

Being empowered in their illness experience, for this author, is political. It not only allows the author to feel an elevation of individualized power, but it calls them to extend that power to those around them experiencing oppression, as well.

Many authors mirrored a perspective of finding strength in a diagnosis. For example, Author 4 explains in their narrative that they were seeking a name for their illness because, for them, "knowledge is [[power]]." However, other authors complicated a linear belief that a diagnosis was an inherent resolution, as it may afford clarity in some aspects, but, as a result, further questions emerge. Author 7 writes that while they were exploring their gender identity, they underwent an exam that indicated ovarian cysts. The author notes:

> This doesn't change my diagnosis or treatment plan but it did provide me with both a sense of validation that PCOS was an accurate diagnosis for me and also an increased sense of uncertainty. How long have I had cysts? When did they develop? Are they stable or growing?

Ultimately, the author questions: "[[Where does this leave me now?]]" In our closing interview, Author 7 elaborated on this narrative moment and explained that receiving a diagnosis was emotionally complex. This is similar to Butler's argument, outlined in Chapter 2, of how a gender identity disorder diagnosis (later renamed in the Diagnostic and Statistical Manual of Mental Disorders as gender dysphoria) can impact individuals in expansive ways. For some, a formal diagnosis could legitimate their health status for access to surgeries, hormonal therapy and insurance coverage. However, naming a disease holds meaning. For some this asserts the body as abnormal which may have dehumanizing implications including calling into question one's gender identity (Butler, *Undoing Gender* 77). The reality is that both experiences might be simultaneously true for most. While Author 7 believes a formal diagnosis can aid a patient in navigating the healthcare system, particularly when seeking referrals to a specialist, diagnostic labels may also be "quite harmful." This harm stems from dynamics of diverse identity intersecting with noninclusive medical diagnostic language, as the author mentions a dissonance created as a nonbinary individual receiving an "assigned female diagnosis" like hyperandrogenism.

Authors discussed the concept of empowerment in relation to an internal, emotional transformation. While the *Click Me* Twine stories tended to swell to an empowered narrative conclusion, this ending typically centred a transformative mindset in order to ultimately accept living with the disease. Author 10 writes:

> At this point in the story, you may be wondering what all these life changes have to do with PCOS. You may think that PCOS is simply a medical issue but for me, it was rooted in this journey of healing and self-discovery. [[As I began to live in my truth, my symptoms started to ease.]]

The Author goes on to describe the most difficult moments of their experience with PCOS, referred to by the author as their personal "dark ages," and concludes that despite the suffering the disease caused them, they believe it was a necessary experience to give them "fuel to figure out what I needed to begin the healing process."

Ultimately, for the author, their experience with the illness has become more bearable because of the lessons they have learned in the process. This is a similar sentiment found in various *Click Me* narratives. In Figure 5.9, Author 9 writes about finding strength in themselves during their fertility journey, explaining: "the person I rely most on is <u>myself</u>." They describe various labourious efforts required when someone is trying to get pregnant, including urinating on ovulation tests and morning temperature checks, ultimately concluding that they are the stable comfort for themselves in difficult times. The author wonders: "Is there an [[end]]?" The following passage explains that there may not be an end to the disease, but there is an end to the author's struggles. While the belief in reaching an emotional state of accepting the disease is expressed in various *Click Me* narratives in different ways, they tend to converge around the concept of transformation. Ultimately, for the authors, to accept the *sickness* is to transform.

Finally, the *Click Me* Twine narratives explored a theme of empowerment through community-building. In particular, authors wrote about the internal

But the person I rely most on is myself. I comfort myself whenever I have to pee at least twice a day to check if I'm ovulating; I give myself a pat in the back if I remember to take my temperature first thing in the morning; and I console myself whenever the second pink line does not show up after waiting for 5 whole minutes.

Sometimes I confuse my sadness with exhaustion. I am tired, emotionally, physically and mentally. But maybe that's it -- I never stop feeling sad, that's why I'm exhausted? At this point, really, I don't care. I just feel tired/sad.

Is there an end?

*Figure 5.9* Screenshot of Author 9's Twine Story.

power that stems from finding kinship with other women and individuals with hyperandrogenism as well as through support from loved ones. Author 3 discusses how social media movements, such as "body positivity or fat acceptance," helped them to develop acceptance of their body as it is. The author notes, through the process of being more open about their hyperandrogenism experience, they discovered that their cousin also has the disease. This bond with their family member has helped the author process how common the disease is and how important it is to reduce the stigma of the diagnosis. Finding empowerment through familial and community bonds was a theme shared by Author 3, as well. In the author's narrative, they consider how cultivating vulnerability by sharing their feelings with loved ones might help the author to cope more effectively with the illness. Ultimately, the author hopes this vulnerability will allow them to "get to the point where I'm not an occasional spectator of the beautiful sunshine on this [[planet…]]… but rather, someone who basks in the sun at any given opportunity." The narrative of transformation, here, is about reframing an internalized belief system, informed through lived experience, that illness impedes living one's life fully and that community support can challenge this.

## Situating Narrative Perspectives

Every *Click Me* Twine formed the same subject position of the narrator through the first-person point of view. In every author's story, the author wrote about their illness experience utilizing the *I* pronoun, rather than *you*.

The textual use of *you* has been theorized extensively by hypertext scholars Alice Bell and Astrid Ensslin ("'Click = Kill': Textual You in Ludic Digital Fiction"; "'I Know What It Was. You Know What It Was': Second-Person Narration in Hypertext Fiction"; "A Reader Response Method Not Just For 'You'"). Assumptions made about the use of the textual *you* as a method to ensure identification by the reader/player would be deeply incomplete. Bell and Ensslin argue that the use of the textual, ambiguous *you* in digital fiction is a highly mediated process between the intentions of the author, the interactivity of the technology and the agency and choices of the reader. Because of this matrix of factors, the use of the textual *you* has the potential to generate complex, distinct outcomes regarding identification with the protagonist of the story. For example, Bell and Ensslin found in a 2019 study that

> readers' negotiation of the various identity positions offered by ambiguous forms of address displayed their tendency to adopt positive identity positions of 'you' but resist negative identity positions by reframing the 'you' as an optional identity that they were expected to psychologically project into.
>
> ("A Reader Response Method not Just for 'You'" 262)

*You*, then, becomes a contentious space for the reader/player to make decisions about where they fit into the story world, in a nonuniform way.

There is a prevalent tradition in Twine writing to use the second-person point of view, where the reader/player becomes a character in the narrative navigating hypertexts that tend to include the *you* pronoun. This convention stems from the common ancestors of Twine storytelling: "game books (choose-your-own-adventure stories), parser-based text adventures (interactive fictions), and hypertext fictions" (Salter and Moulthrop 139). For example, in Anna Anthropy's *Queers in Love at the End of the World*, the reader/player becomes the protagonist of the story: "it's just the two of you together. You have ten seconds, but there's so much you want to do: [[kiss]] her, [[hold]] her, [[take]] her hand, [[tell]] her." When the *Click Me* authors centre the first-person perspective, it could be argued that they foreground the experience of themselves as the author rather than that of the reader/player. This breaks with the interactive fiction tradition that tends to explore the choices and beliefs of the reader/player, designed by the author.

A simplistic analysis of this phenomenon might suggest that *Click Me* authors overwhelmingly chose to build a Twine that embodied a narrative story rather than a game-like structure. However, this phenomenon is inserting itself into a larger, relatively unresolved scholarly debate around formalism and the game-ness of literary hypertext. Salter and Moulthrop argue that

> At a certain point in the early history of digital fiction, it was fashionable to accuse them of debasing literature (see most notoriously Birkerts). Nonetheless, figures associated with hypertext, such as Joyce, Shelley Jackson, and John McDaid, have been identified mainly as fiction writers. (140)

However, as Ensslin argues in *Literary Gaming* (2014), game and story are not distinct categories, and the boundaries of one may seep into the other. Ultimately, this is what Twine is. Twine is self-aware of this inability to pin it down. Chapbook, one of Twine's built-in story formats, has an official GitHub guide that includes the following note:

> Keeping in the spirit of vexing formalists who prefer clear boundaries, this guide calls the things you'll create with Chapbook stories and the people who you share them with players, but you shouldn't infer anything from this usage. Please make strange things with Twine and Chapbook.

This tradition of using Twine to make strange is embodied in the *Click Me* stories in expansive ways. Perhaps some authors may view their first-person narrative as a game, while others see theirs as a piece of literature. Others may identify with both or neither. As Salter and Moulthrop argue, "Twine inherits this contradiction. It is structurally familiar and formally suggests so many antecedents that it does not at first glance appear transgressive–and yet it transgresses and transforms" (26).

Rather than assert the extent of the game-ness or narrative-ness the authors' Twines embody because of the first-person perspective, it may be more productive to grapple with why this style was popular. An obvious reason would be an expectation the authors interpreted from the writing prompt to explore their subjective experience. Although the *Click Me* authors did spend time in the module reading other example Twine games for inspiration, all of which were written in the second-person point of view. This, theoretically, would also have the potential to sway writing style. There is not enough information to analyze why the *Click Me* authors chose the first-person perspective in their writing, however, there may be a similar impact from this choice. Where conventional Twine games appear to foreground the choices of the reader through the second-person point of view, the *Click Me* authors used Twine to centre their own subjectivity.

One author, Author 9, while still using the first-person perspective, creates a metalepsis, or the transgression of narrative levels, by acknowledging the reader/player. A passage of this author's story reads: "If you chose to click this link, then hello, I want to tell you something more than my *PCOS-related problems*." This is the sole narrative in the study that includes the use of a "you" pronoun, however, the author still employs a first-person perspective. The second-person pronoun is employed in a self-reflexive way to draw attention to both the reader reading and the author writing the story. A later passage reads: "I hope you also find a way to deal with your own struggles, no matter how big or small they are; *don't be so hard on yourself*, we all have issues." Empathy, particularly empathy for the reader/player, has sat at the crux of the game-ness/narrative-ness Twine debate for years. Salter and Moulthrop explain how, in response to critics of Twine who challenge a lack of game-like objectives, authors such as Leigh Alexander and Raph Koster raise the question of empathy. Alexander wonders how understanding another human is not considered a challenge and Koster argues that games conveying empathy for the reader/player rather than the other way around are much more difficult to design (Salter and Moulthrop 23). Although Author 9's narrative deviates from the others in the study by including reference to the reader/player, the narrative creates a similar impact where the reader/player is hailed as an audience, solely to hear the experience of the author.

The narrative subject positions formed by the *Click Me* authors enact and restrict moments for action in different ways. However, all the Twines build a formulaic trajectory for the author's agency. The stories begin with setting a scene for a lack of agency for the author and, as the narrative processes, the author is granted or restricted agency through their narrative encounter with other subjects, objects and forces. The subject position of the author is framed initially as powerless, with oppositional forces enacting oppression onto the body. These oppositional forces are vast but include puberty as violence onto the body, the author's own body as a character, fatphobic physicians, the opinions of the mother, the labour of fertility, or the physical pain of hair removal practices. All these forces work together to restrict the agency of the author. However, the *Click Me* Twines collectively shift the narrative tone, through encounters with other forces, to grant moments of action for the author as the story progresses. For example, narratives facilitate agency for the author through encounters with alternative medicine practices, talk therapy, formal diagnosis or knowledge accumulation. This becomes significant as the *Click Me* authors did not frame the inherent embodiment of hyperandrogenism as restricting agency but as how the illness is taken up culturally. Logically, it follows that moments granting action for the author did not come from alleviating symptoms of the illness but through encounters with cultural forces that pushed back against illness stigma.

### Narrative Interaction with Outside Agents

The *Click Me* authors chose distinct and meaningful ways to intersect their narratives with external texts, authors and readers. Most notably, this was done through choices authors made around considering differing reader/player experiences and foregrounding traditionally authoritative informational resources versus less authoritative sources. In one narrative, written by Author 12, the author takes into consideration how various reader/players may experience their story by including a content warning. The opening passage of this author's story includes a line that reads: "*Note: My story comes with a warning because they all include themes, which may cause a strong reaction in women with similar experiences." The author, in this disclaimer, is grappling with how the experience of some readers, namely women with hyperandrogenism, may be different than others because of the potential of a strong emotional reaction to the narrative content. This content warning, written by the author, speaks to how narrative meaning becomes altered through the text's dialectic with other agents, including reader/players. It becomes important for this author to convey the complexity of the reader experience and how the intended meaning, in their story, may shift with each unique reader experience.

While the *Click Me* narratives, in many ways, undermined the authority of traditional pillars of knowledge, namely the normative healthcare system, simultaneously these same narratives upheld other forms of authoritative knowledge. For example, Author 10 incorporates a statistic from The World Health Organization that describes how often PCOS is diagnosed across the world. Author 12 includes an external URL link to a diet challenge. The author writes: "I am now more determined than ever to get PCOS out of my life. I did the 30 Day PCOS Diet Challenge with Kym Cambell, her website is https://www.smartfertilitychoices.com/." These choices made by the authors to incorporate external texts into their narrative is a productive action that further shapes the meaning of their story. Similarly, in Author 11's narrative, the author shares the Oxford English Dictionary definition of the term shame as "noun a painful feeling of humiliation or distress caused by the consciousness of wrong or foolish behaviour. verb (of a person, action, or situation) make (someone) feel ashamed." This dialectic with an external text generates additional, complex meaning in the narrative of the author.

The definition of shame Author 11 chooses to include reinforces the belief that the origin of shame is the fault of the individual. The definition situates the root of the emotion as "the consciousness of wrong or foolish behaviour" rather than a consciousness of how the world treats individuals based on social stigma. This interpretation of the term alters the meaning, or rather, makes shame mean the fault of the author. This paints the meaning of the author's narrative in various ways. The definition of shame is the opening passage in this narrative. Once the reader/player moves on from this passage, they are confronted with anecdotes from the author that centre the abnormal body, symptoms and feelings of inadequacy. Most of these passages loop back to the opening passage about shame. For example, in a subsequent passage (analyzed in a previous section of this chapter) the author describes how infertility affects their relationship, “I know the suffering is not just my own. My spouse, excited as he was at the first positive also feels the pain of each negative test as well. Sometimes I think he blames me. And I don’t fault him on that. I blame [[me]] too.” When the reader/player selects the [[me]] hypertext, they are looped back to the definition of shame. Not only does the author create a literal and figurative link between their illness experiences and the emotion of shame, but, reinforced by this textual understanding of shame, blame is situated with the author. This is an example of how external texts intersecting with the author narratives expanded, stretched, shifted and deconstructed narrative meaning.

While most external texts that authors engaged with in their narratives could be considered traditionally authoritative, one author challenged this pattern. Author 7 built a Twine narrative that centred knowledge dissemination where, before the author wrote about their experience with a particular issue, they chose to define and contextualize the issue with external links to information sources. In some cases, the author chooses to link to traditionally authoritative sources such as the Mayo Clinic or the Migraine Institute. The author includes descriptions of various symptoms and informs the reader/player that “Hyperandrogenism should be considered for anyone who presents with hirsutism, menstrual disturbance, or central obesity during puberty.” The author provides a definition of hirsutism including the phonetic pronunciation and a URL to a page about the condition on the Mayo Clinic’s website. While the author upholds traditionally authoritative knowledge in some ways, they also make stark decisions to challenge it by incorporating alternative sources.

For example, the author writes about their experience as a nonbinary individual. In this discussion, they define and explain to the reader/player the differences between the terms sex, gender and gender identity. The author notes: “It’s common for people to confuse sex, gender, and gender identity. But they’re actually all different things.” In a later passage, the author includes the following line of code:

> <img src="https://www.genderbread.org/resource/genderbread-person-v4-0" width="600" height="800" alt="Use it Online">.

This line produces an infographic of The Gender Bread Person, a popular teaching resource created by Hues, a global justice collective of artists, educators, and activists co-created in 2017 by Sam Killermann. This teaching resource is less mainstream than, say, the Mayo Clinic, and it produces the sentiment that the author is committed to teaching the reader/player about not only their illness experience but also the political ideologies that intersect with their story.

In our closing interview, Author 7 reflected on incorporating concept definitions into literary hypertext, noting:

> I think in storytelling, we often struggle with needing to give like background or definitions and things like that. So that tool just allows you to kind of incorporate those without, I think, taking away from like the narrative of the story.

The author is highlighting Twine's ability to compartmentalize narrative pieces into separate passages, which, by creating a system of hypertextual division, ironically for the author, allowed for increased narrative flow. This is because informative resources and definitions related to the narrative could supplement the story without creating a stark intervention. This system of hypertextual division allows hypertext authors the ability to populate their narratives with contextual information similar to footnotes, in ways that enhance and enrich the flow of the storytelling rather than detracting from it. As Author 7 sees it, readers can engage deeper and more meaningfully with the narrative through the supplemental contextual information which, ultimately, may support the pedagogical goals of some Twines.

## Narrative Affirmation and Erasure

In reflecting on the analysis of the *Click Me* narrative themes, insight emerges around what is generally affirmed and erased in the discursive framing of the authors' Twines. Collectively, the *Click Me* narratives affirm that a female body that experiences masculinizing symptoms is abnormal. This abnormality renders the body in need of control, deciphering and strenuous maintenance. The default in the abnormal body runs the risk of seeping into the author's psyche as well, ultimately rooting the abnormal body in emotional bankruptcy. In turn, narratives affirm that bodily abnormality is undesirable because of its relationality with outside agents rather than an inherent undesirability. It is in the author's encounters with other people, institutions and social systems that make their bodies undesirable, not the neutral embodiment of symptoms. This turning to the cultural take-up of disease as the culprit of facilitating suffering, rather than embodied symptoms, is reminiscent of Couser's novel category of a counterhegemonic and postcolonial challenging narrative style known as the rhetoric of emancipation discussed in Chapter 1. These narratives are inherently political in nature, according to Couser, where the rhetoric of emancipation is attuned to the political struggle of identity for disabled people. These narratives focus less on eradicating symptoms and more on institutional recognition of the humanity and rights of those with disabilities (Couser, *Signifying Bodies* 47).

For the *Click Me* authors, moments of Couser's notion of emancipation looked like reflection on dehumanizing experiences in the healthcare system and naming moments of body-based injustice. The *Click Me* narratives affirm that illness is a personal journey of growth where, in order to heal therapeutically, the patient must resolve a perception of emotional bankruptcy, gain knowledge, receive a formal diagnosis and locate a community of support. Finally, the *Click Me* Twines affirm the belief that encounters in the normative healthcare system are generally dehumanizing, subjugating, or violating. Female physicians, for many authors, generally acted as characters who challenged this trend by making authors feel validated, heard and understood. Overall, authors affirmed alternative methods as an effective response to their illness, not because of a measured reduction of symptoms, but because of producing a greater sense of well-being.

By reinforcing particular belief systems, the *Click Me* narratives work to erase various counter-discourses. Most notably, upholding traditional biomedical approaches, a sense of contentment with the abnormal, and questioning the category of abnormality was erased. While the *Click Me* Twine stories tended to challenge the omnipotence of the normative healthcare system, this led to an erasure of upholding a biomedical model of illness that, some argue, rejects a holistic approach to treatment. Generally, the *Click Me* Twines did not approach the concept of the abnormal body as positive or even neutral. In the same vein, there were few narrative moments when authors explicitly questioned abnormality as a category or challenged dichotomies of healthy and ill or normal and pathological. It is important to mention this outcome without value judgment. These findings do not lend to an analytical interpretation that questioning these dichotomies would be good or bad. This was an expected outcome as the *Click Me* authors were invited to share their stories of illness. Explored in depth in previous chapters of this book, the ways in which illness and pathology intersect with gender identity are highly complex and produce significant, meaningful impacts on the lives and well-being of individuals

## Works Cited

Anthropy, Anna. *Queers in Love at the End of the World*. itch.io, 12 March 2016, https://w.itch.io/end-of-the-world

Bell, Alice, and Astrid Ensslin. "'Click = Kill': Textual You in Ludic Digital Fiction." *Storyworlds: A Journal of Narrative Studies*, vol. 4, 2012, pp. 49–73.

Anthropy, Anna. "'I Know What It Was. You Know What It Was': Second-Person Narration in Hypertext Fiction." *Narrative*, vol. 19, no. 3, 2011, pp. 311–329.

Anthropy, Anna, et al. "A Reader Response Method Not Just For 'You'." *Language and Literature*, vol. 28, no. 3, 2019, pp. 241–262.

Butler, Judith. *Bodies That Matter: On the Discursive Limits of "Sex"*. Routledge, 2011.

Butler, Judith. *Undoing Gender*. Routledge, 2004, pp. 40–56.
"Chapbook Guide." *Github*, https://klembot.github.io/chapbook/guide/index.html. Accessed 5 December 2022.
Couser, G. Thomas. *Signifying Bodies: Disability in Contemporary Life Writing*. University of Michigan Press, 2009.
Ensslin, Astrid. *Literary Gaming*. MIT Press, 2014.
Frank, Arthur W. *The Wounded Storyteller: Body, Illness, and Ethics*, 2nd ed. The University of Chicago Press, 2013.
Perram, Megan. "Illness of the Gendered Body, Freud's *The Uncanny*, and 'being-in-the-world'." *Canadian Review of Comparative Literature*, vol. 46, no. 4, 2019, pp. 587–600.
Puar, Jasbir K. "'I Would Rather Be a Cyborg Than a Goddess': Becoming-Intersectional in Assemblage Theory." *philoSOPHIA: A Journal of Continental Feminism*, vol. 2, no. 1, 2012, pp. 49–66.
Salter, Anastasia, and Stuart Moulthrop. *Twining*. Amherst College Press, 2021.

# 6 How Code Makes Meaning or Mapping the Illness Narrative

### Using Twine

While the previous chapter explored the narrative concepts constructed through the *Click Me* Twines and their affective relations with the world, this chapter will tackle the technology. How does hypertext make meaning? Even if hypertext holds the promise of therapeutic benefit, how accessible and user-friendly, really, is the Twine software? Ultimately, how does this practice of building a Twine differ from writing the story of the self on a piece of paper or in a Word document? What makes hypertext something to be excited about? This chapter will trouble the promise of hypertext accessibility through the lens of capacity, which may take many forms: physical, emotional, mental, financial. It will explore how code makes meaning and how the simple coding element choices made by the *Click Me* authors contribute to larger sociopolitical discourse, generating oceans of meaning beyond the confines of the Twine program. The chapter will then outline the most compelling finding of this research which is how authors spoke about the therapeutic potential of using literary hypertext technology to write illness narratives. The *Click Me* authors explored, in different ways, the concept of using the digital features of Twine to visually map out their experiences and manually organize them by hyperlinking passages. This process allowed them to find a structure that they felt was best suited for personal reflection. Finally, this chapter will address the ultimate question of therapeutic value. It will find that authors reiterated a common belief: writing an illness narrative in literary hypertext does not hold a comprehensive curative effect on the self but can offer a valuable opportunity to reflect on past experiences. Authors concluded that these stories need to be shared with healthcare practitioners who treat individuals with hyperandrogenism to serve as a tool for teaching about experiences of the disease, ultimately to inspire more ethical and comprehensive care.

The *Click Me* authors ultimately found that Twine was impactful as a tool to visually map out their experiences, and manually organize them by

DOI: 10.4324/9781003646921-6

hyperlinking passages, to find a structure that was best suited for therapeutic reflection. While Twine has a sociohistorical legacy as a tool of resistance, the way the *Click Me* authors highlighted that accessibility is complex. Power relations, according to authors, can monopolize capacity, particularly the capacity to sit down and learn a new technology for writing. Ultimately, authors reinforced that engaging in authoring a single hypertext narrative cannot—and is not intended to—have purely curative outcomes in relation to emotional wellbeing. However, what was beneficial for authors in the writing process was reflecting on past experiences, which led to new vantage points to better understand emotions, the establishment of a connection to the self, and validation of experiences of injustice. Authors concluded by affirming that the true transformative potential for literary hypertext illness narratives about hyperandrogenism would be as a teaching tool for health-care providers and the wider community to learn about the experience of hyperandrogenism. The summarized finding of the *Click Me* project, in response to the research question is as follows: individuals with hyperandrogenism can use literary hypertext to write illness narratives that build positive relationships between themselves and the world by engaging with various themes and software features to visually map and organize experiences into a structure best suited for reflection, both for individual therapy and for institutional pedagogy.

In closing interviews, authors overwhelmingly spoke to the accessibility of the Twine software in various ways. Most notably, authors discussed Twine as user-friendly and straightforward to learn when following the steps outlined in the *Click Me* module. Author 11, for example, explained how the module gave them all the information they required to build their story, although, they chose to Google additional information to expand the scope of their project. Author 4 noted: "I thought it was very, very easy to use. And that tutorial was awesome. So that is all I needed. And then I was on my way." However, the accessibility of Twine was predicated on the assumption of time. Authors explained that although Twine was eventually straightforward to use, it took them some time to get to a place where they were prepared to write. Being appropriately prepared for the *Click Me* authors looked like having the time to concentrate on the module instructions and the emotional or mental capacity to write about difficult experiences. Author 11 explained that they initially were struggling to start the module: "But I was also like, at work and I was distracted. So the second time I attempted it was, it was much easier to grasp, I guess, when I didn't have the same distractions."

Beyond distractions and mental capacity, some authors explained that Twine initially felt too daunting. One author mentioned that they felt nervous to start the tutorial because of a reference to coding I made in our screening interview. They were pleasantly surprised at how user-friendly the software was after they did begin the *Click Me* module. Author 9 shared that engaging in the module's storyboarding exercise, which asked authors to free write, among other tasks, on a physical sheet of paper, was imperative to their success in completing their Twine story. They explained that having a physical outline of their story before they started to engage with the more complex software of Twine allowed them to focus on learning the program without being overwhelmed with brainstorming a narrative topic at the same time. Another author explained that the inherent structure of Twine was actually less overwhelming than sitting down to write a narrative on a physical sheet of paper. For this author, the structure of literary hypertext was more inviting because it breaks down the mass bulk of text into smaller, more digestible sections. This is a compelling perspective because it speaks to an issue that many writers discuss, of feeling paralyzed at the start of the writing process because a blank, white screen or paper reflects a sense of absence that needs to be filled. Twine, on the other hand, allows the author to build the narrative in smaller, progressive steps.

One author found the software too complex. I ended up working with this author to build their narrative into the software for them. In our closing interview, they explained

> I'm old, right? [laughs] So, for me to learn, like new stuff, I have to do it all the time for my job. So when it came to this, I was a little bit like, overwhelmed with the like program.

This author shares that despite not completing the literary hypertext design portion of the study independently, they still felt the experience of writing their illness narrative was impactful. The author believed they would have been successful if they were able to learn Twine in an in-person session. Although this was one author's experience, this is a critical finding of this research. While some individuals may feel empowered through online pedagogy, others may be more successful through an in-person environment.

Although there was a strong and clear consensus amongst authors that Twine was easy to use and learn, there was discussion of various minor technical issues. One author noted that accessing Twine on their phone made some text unreadable and switching to a laptop fixed the issue. A couple of authors shared frustrations they had with publishing their stories to file, a built-in feature of Twine's that allows authors to download their stories as an HTML file on their desktop. While the *Click Me* module outlines the steps of this process, it fails to offer troubleshooting techniques to account for different computer settings. Further, various, beginner CSS and HTML codes were available for authors including codes to alter text alignment, size and style, but most authors either chose not to include any code or simply alter text colours. Author 11 explained in our closing interview that after they played the example Twine games in the module, they wanted to replicate some of the stylistic features in their own story. However, the author notes, "I was trying to figure that out. But in the interest of my time too like, I just didn't have time, but it would have been cool to kind of customize it a little more."

Author 16 explained that by manipulating the colour codes of their Twine's text and background, they were unable to make their narrative "look pretty" and ultimately felt that the story "looked ugly." The author did not elaborate on their intentions or what "pretty" and "ugly" meant to them, but this comment struck me during the interview and continues to resonate as I write this text. I am curious about the inherent expectations of aesthetics in relation to art that the *Click Me* authors—or any of us, for that matter—might hold. There is an assumption, at times, that the art we create should be beautiful or visually pleasant. I wonder though, why beauty in art may be important to this particular *Click Me* author? Why is it important to most of us who create art? What would it mean if this author's story was, in fact, visually "ugly"? Are there internalized connections that we cannot yet see that link between the self and the art we create? This is a fascinating inquiry to examine in future research along with barriers to access around computer programming, especially for marginalized people living with illness.

## How Code Makes Meaning

In her 2004 article "Print is Flat, Code is Deep," N. Katherine Hayles argues "We can no longer afford to pretend that texts are immaterial or that text on screen is the same as text in print. The immateriality of the text has ceased to be a useful or even a viable fiction" (86–87). Hayles' work in hypertext theory highlights the significance of accounting for the embodied materiality of code and how this materiality makes meaning. Meaning in literary hypertext is formed through a matrix of factors including the relationality of physical artefacts of the digital text, discourse and content, and the encounters between readers and authors. In the *Click Me* project, authors chose to incorporate CSS and HTML code, for example, in various ways that contributed to the meaning-making of their Twine stories. In particular, authors used colour, alignment, size and text style code to design the look of their narratives.

At the time of the study, authors used the Twine 2.3.8 release in the Harlowe 3.1.0 story format. This story format sets default colours. The background of a Twine story is black, the text is white, and the hyperlinks are blue. These default colours can be altered through colour codes that target the HTML, a process that the module explains to authors. While text colour can be altered through manipulating RGB values, HSL values or hexadecimal code, the module outlines the most simplistic, yet limited, option of inserting the colour name into pre-existing CSS. CSS specifies basic colour names that attribute to what is known as keywords. From here, properties in CSS can take these keywords and ultimately set the text and background colours. Authors were given a snippet of CSS to insert into their Story Stylesheet and shown how to replace the colour of the Twine's text, background and hyperlinks. Of the five authors who changed the default background colour of their Twines, most (three) changed the default black background to white with black text. This was an interesting finding because the authors actively incorporated colour codes into their stories in order to reproduce a rather familiar digital appearance. White background with black text is a standard colour combination used for various websites, applications and digital writing documents. Rather than choose to challenge assumed expectations around how a digital narrative document should look, authors chose to reproduce this.

This choice may have been made for various reasons, including the fact that a white background with black text may be presumed as the most readable combination. Richardson et al. conducted a review of the literature on colour and contrast in e-learning and found that luminance contrast, which measures the difference between the brightness of foreground elements relative to the background, was the most critical factor in determining the legibility of text and symbols (658). Richardson et al. note that in a seminal study conducted, Murch (1987) found that black text on a white background was widely deemed by writers as a legible contrast. However, this study found alternative colour combinations as more legible including black text on a green background and blue text on a white background (Richardson et al. 659). In addition, this study finds that Harlowe's default colours (white text, blue hyperlinks and black background) were found to be equally as legible as black text and a white background (Richardson et al. 659). Following a review of the literature, Richardson et al. ultimately conclude that accessibility in relation to digital reading is highly complex and goes beyond colour contrast including text size and font. The authors note that "These findings indicate that visually impaired users have different needs. For all users, the interplay of text style and background color can have other effects—beyond readability—which can influence learning" (Richardson et al. 660). There is perhaps a path emerging to argue that the *Click Me* authors' choice to replicate the colours of a standard digital writing document, rather than the expansive colour palettes typically found in video games, speaks to perceptions around favouring narrative-ness over gameness. However, this argument would be too simplistic and not informed by the findings. It is beyond the scope of this research to study how colour choices were made by authors, however, understanding why a standard colour contrast was popular would be important for future research.

Ensslin argues in *Canonizing Hypertext* (2007) that "With respect to hypermedia, authors employ images, animation, film and sound to create additional layers of meaning, which correlate to textual meaning in various ways” (21). Several authors chose to include images in their Twines, including selfies, memes, infographics and a motivational quote set on an image of a summiting mountaineer. One author chose to include images of themself in their Twine, showing what they call a “before” and “after” picture. Subverting the typical tradition through which content is labelled with this language, mainly for marking weight loss progress, this author merely captures their smiling face in both images. The alt attribute, which specifies an alternate text for an image if the image cannot be displayed, is labelled by the author as: <alt=“Before picture of seeing a Naturopathic”>. The author describes exploring multiple healthcare avenues to address their illness, to no avail. They finally decide to visit a naturopathic doctor and feel a sense of hope. Sitting in the waiting room for this initial consultation, the author writes “my husband pulls out my Iphone and I tell him to take a [[before picture]].” Later in the narrative, after the author has experienced positive results from their naturopathic treatment, they write: “[[Here is a current picture of me]] shows that I am feeling better than I did when I was taking birth control at the begining [sic] of this very wild journey.” For the reader/player of this author’s story, there is little difference between the person in the images. Their hair is longer in the after shot and they are standing presumably outdoors as the background is washed out from sunlight. Perhaps the lack of a stark visual difference indicates that the transformation for the author was beyond the body.

Style and colour codes were used by the *Click Me* authors in diverse ways. Mainly, when authors did choose to incorporate style codes, they employed them in ways that transformed their narratives into a visual experience where the colour, size, style and spacing of the text produced narrative meaning. For example, Author 3 describes a scene where they are looking at themselves in the mirror. One passage reads: “Except all I see reflected is just me.” The word “me,” however, is set apart from the rest of the phrase. It sits alone on a lower line, right-aligned, enlarged and in bold red colour. This is a simple, yet striking, use of basic stylistic code employed by the author to generate an embodied representation of the self as exiled, alone or, perhaps, obtrusive. The author ends their narrative by describing the methods of “acceptance”, “understanding” and “empowerment” that allowed them to come to a place of contentment with their body. The last passage replays the moment of the opening scene, however, this time “me” looks different. In Figure 6.1, the text is still enlarged and right-aligned, however, it is no longer in bold red, but a familiar black that is uniform throughout the textual narrative. This stylistic choice made by the author creates a neat bookend that captures a sentiment that the author still may struggle with their illness, but they have found small ways to accept themselves. Author 16 creates a similar visual in their closing passage. The author writes several phrases that ponder the possibility of an illness cure or relief for the symptoms of the body, such

My condition is just one part of me.

Mirror, mirror on the wall...

I gaze into the mirror.

All I see reflected is just

**me.**

*Figure 6.1* Screenshot C of Author 3's Twine Story.

as "Maybe next month the number will budge," or "Maybe the skin will get lighter." Each of these statements begin with the word "maybe." The final line of the narrative is a single "maybe" standing alone and emboldened. This simple design choice effectively creates a sentiment for the reader/player that the author is suspended in the maybe, not here nor there, but the unknown.

Using style codes to organize texts and hyperlinks into a visual experience was a common strategy used by the *Click Me* authors. In Figure 6.2, Author 4 is listing the symptoms of their illness and the emotions these symptoms produce. Instead of listing the symptoms in a typical way—with uniform size, in a single line, and left-aligned—the author arranges these elements to form a visual scene. Each symptom is placed in a different column and on a separate line. As the reader progresses through the symptoms, the text grows larger and more menacing. For me, this passage resembles the motion of descending a staircase, leading the reader deeper into the depths of the illness. Similarly, Author 3 centres the uncomfortable experience of hair removal in their narrative. In one passage, the author describes the painful sensation of removing facial hair by a threading method, noting: "The taut thread grates across my skin, taking small hairs at a slow, painful one strand at a time." The latter five words of the statement, however, are set apart. The author sets each word on a single line. Double spacing encloses each word in isolation. As the reader/player you are forced to halt, searing in each word as if a single strand of hair is ripped in sequence from your skin as well. This intentional, affective use of style codes by Author 3, and other *Click Me* authors, is a method of immersion. Akin to poetry, the reader/player is called

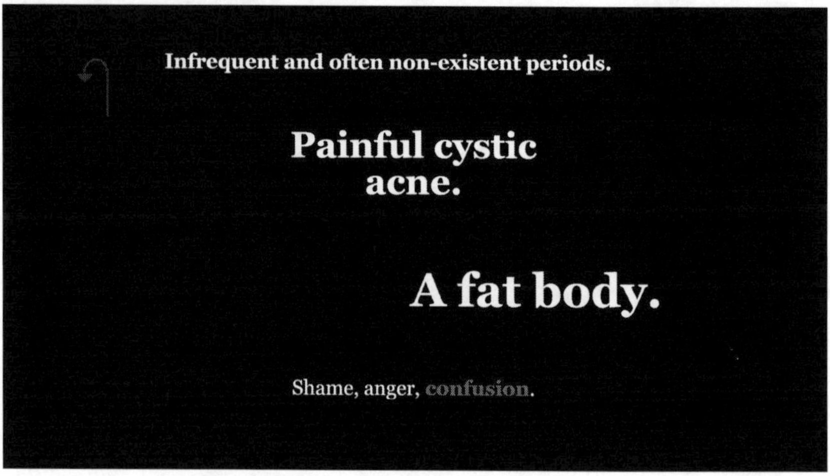


*Figure 6.2* Screenshot of Author 4's Twine Story.

on to engage with the text in more visceral ways that work to enhance the storytelling experience overall.

**Designing Hypertext**

The *Click Me* authors, in closing interviews, discussed the significance of their choices regarding hyperlinks within their narratives. They explained that text positioned to be a hyperlink was an intentional choice made and this text was ultimately meant to stand as a focal point to emphasize key moments or themes in their narratives. Author 4 describes that they choose to hyperlink text in order to cultivate a specific tone for their narrative:

> it was almost like I was able to remove myself out of the situation, but also write about myself, but kind of almost like, on a different plane, because then I was sort of looking back to see how was I feeling. And how are those feelings [are] important to the story and, and the tone. And then which words then would be the best to hyperlink to the next…the next page.

Ultimately, the hyperlink text that the *Click Me* authors built shaped the meaning produced by their stories.

For the reader/player, the hyperlink text choice marks the text as meaningful to the narrative by inherently signalling the progression of the plot. Hypertext is a door that leads the reader/player to the next passage and therefore embodies meaning beyond textual discourse. For example, in

Author 16's narrative, they discuss the emotional impacts of culturally negotiating a body perceived as abnormal. The author writes: "But how does anyone look past the weight?" The next passage reads: "Because I don't know if I can sometimes. [[Well]]." The final word is set apart from the other text on a different line. The hyperlink function renders the word blue, in contrast to the white colouring of the subsequent text in the passage. This choice made by the author to emphasize the word [[Well]], through alignment and hyperlinking, swells the meaning of this simple passage in expansive ways. The word "well" is an unassuming, ambiguous word that holds enormous potential for interpretation. "Well" encompasses a range of emotions such as exasperation, exhaustion, dismay and hopelessness. It is a slippery term that is difficult to pin down. It can be an exclamation of surprise, anger, resignation or relief. But it can also mean the absence of illness. There is an expectation, in the context of literary hypertext, that if the reader/player clicks on [[Well]], they will be brought to a passage that connects physically and thematically to the hyperlink text. The linked passage in Author 16's story signals defeat, resignation and a loss of hope: "I guess this isn't the moment. Maybe next month it will be." In the case of Author 16, when a simple word is chosen as the hyperlink, it works to propel meaning beyond the boundaries of a linear story. The opinions for creating meaning through hypertext design do not end here.

As discussed in Chapter 4, the authors were introduced to three Twine story structures in the *Click Me* module, which I name as a *forward path*, a *weaving path* and *multiple paths*. A forward path is when the story moves the reader/player through a linear plot progression. There is only a single hypertext option in each passage for the reader/player in this scenario, however, this structure is useful for designing a uniform reading experience. A weaving path branches the narrative into two or multiple hypertext passages but ultimately comes back to a single path. The final narrative structure, multiple paths, incorporates a multitude of hypertext paths for the reader/player to follow. In this structure, each path may describe a different plot and narrative conclusion. The module explains that multiple paths may be more complex and time-consuming to build, but they have the potential to be a generative method to "play through" different scenarios or dream up alternative ways things could have been in relation to the illness experience. As depicted in Figure 6.3, each story structure was ultimately built by a *Click Me* author, however, a weaving path was the dominant choice. There are many possible reasons why this path may have been popular for authors, including the time constraints of the workshop.

The *Click Me* authors tended to utilize a weaving path, and at times multiple paths, to design a narrative loop within their stories. Narrative loops built into the authors' stories included hyperlinks that bring the reader/player back to engage with a previous passage. The cyclical loop was

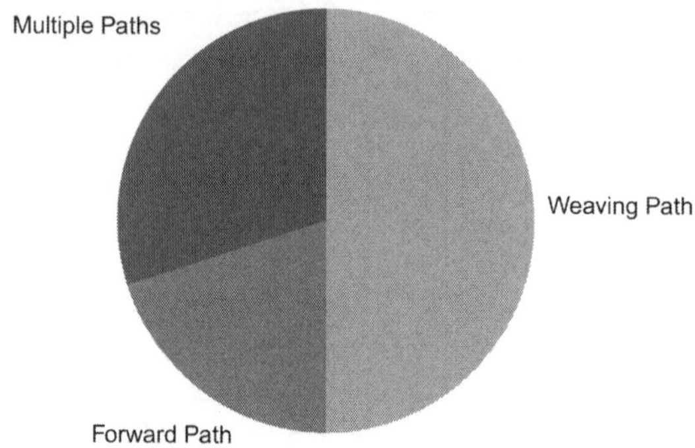


*Figure 6.3* Pie Chart of Path Choice Found in Author Narratives.

discussed by authors in closing interviews as an effective method to personify the experience of their illness. Some authors used the cyclical loop to convey the labour of maintaining the normality of the body. Through various hair removal practices, for example, one author designed a loop where the reader/player becomes stuck in a continuous cycle of hair growth and removal. Other authors discussed negative mental health circuits they were able to build into their Twine narrative. Author 11 explained that they built a loop centred around returning to the feeling of shame in their narrative to mirror their illness experience. They explain: "there's times where it's like, yeah, like things are finally going, it's good to be hopeful. And then you just, it all goes back to the beginning."

Author 16 discussed their illness journey as dominated by a feeling of being enclosed within a loop where they would make efforts to change their body only to be met with stagnation. This bodily stasis would trigger a cycle of harmful thoughts. This author was able to map this circuit in their Twine story. The opening passage notes the amount of work the author has put in to "get this weight off" followed by several hypertext options of actions the reader/player can take. Each option you click will loop you back to the opening passage with a single hypertext that reads: "[[So why won't the scale move?]]." The author contextualizes the cyclical loop they designed, explaining: "this really does affect your mental health… if I'm doing all these things and my body isn't allowing me to love it the way I need to, to be healthy then like, how am I supposed to love it?" This design structure effectively plays with the idea of choice for the reader/player. While it appears the narrative offers hyperlink options to move the story through a chosen plot, ultimately, the reader/player is always looped back to the beginning. This reinforces an oppressive feeling of an illness that has power over the life of the author.

Using a weaving path to play with the idea of reader choice was a popular strategy for the *Click Me* authors in different ways. While some authors, like

Author 12, designed an illusion of choice, other authors foregrounded the agency of the reader/player in the narrative. This juxtaposition was most clearly marked in the stories of Authors 5 and 9. In one passage of Author 5's narrative, the story splits into a weaving path. This is a stark deviation from the precedent of a forward path established in previous passages of the narrative. The author writes: "It's a tough feeling. But on others [sic] days, I feel [[empowered]] [[strong]] [[resilient]]." This narrative split seemingly offers the reader/player a moment of choice. Which adjective will they select? Whichever path is taken, if the reader/player decides to move backward in the narrative via the undo arrow, they will see the sentiment of agency crumble. All three options yield the same passage that reads: "And those are the days that push me to go outside and see the [[light]]."

This strategy to create an illusion of choice is countered by other authors. For example, in Author 9's narrative, the author gives the reader/player the ultimate choice in the opening passage. The reader/player can choose to embark on the lengthy and emotional path described by the author as: "a [[story]] about PCOS-induced infertility." There is a different option, however, sitting beneath the initial line of text. This path, described as [[different topic]], will bring the reader/player to the end of the narrative. Without experiencing any of the passages throughout the Twine, the reader/player moves to the end of the story where the author writes: "If you chose to click this link, then hello, I want to tell you something more than my *PCOS-related problems*." In this final passage, the author outlines what they are grateful for in their life. This is the ultimate design for hypertext choice because it allows the reader/player to decide to not read through the author's illness experience at all.

Returning to Salter and Moulthrop's analysis, they offer three terms to describe the linking strategies of a literary hypertext author. *Navigational* linking identifies the movement of a character or point of view through a story world space, *procedural* linking uses described action as an anchor, and *conversational* linking relies on responsive speech as the anchor of the hypertext (Salter and Moulthrop 69). These terms categorize the narrative text that authors choose to become hypertext links. For the *Click Me* project, all three linking strategies were utilized by authors in their narratives, including a fourth and fifth category, coded as *other* linking and *dead-end* linking.

*Other* linking was an additional category included to capture hypertexts that failed to fit neatly into Salter and Moulthrop's analysis. For example, the hypertext link "[[I've been giving myself the time and space to create healing modalities]]" was coded as *other* linking. Although perhaps this hypertext link fits most closely to *procedural* linking because it details an action of the persona, it fails to embody the definition offered by Salter and Moulthrop. The authors describe *procedural* linking as "where the anchoring text describes an action involving the persona: 'You shut the door';

'The ostrich says nothing'; 'The Twinebot emits another burst of story'" (Salter and Moulthrop 69). The difference in the action detailed by the example hypertext and the definition is that the former fails to offer the reader/player a sense of choice. The reader/player, in this example, is not choosing a hypertext action of the persona to further the plot, this was the only hypertext link in the passage that describes a reflection on the action by the author.

*Dead-end* linking was a category included in the coding of the narratives to capture a path that has no further links. Most stories included at least one *dead end* link, to produce the "final" passage of their narratives, however, *dead-end* linking was utilized by authors in additional ways. Most notably, authors used *dead-end* linking in various passages of their story to create a sense of a lack of options where the only path forward is to move backwards. For example, Author 4 includes a passage detailing the various symptoms of hyperandrogenism. They write: "Do you have the following symptoms? [[Adult acne]] [[Irregular periods]] [[Sporadic fluctuations in weight]]." The reader/player must select one of these symptoms to move forward in the Twine, however, the first two symptoms are a *dead-end* link. Once the reader/player is taken to the next passage, they are confronted with a single word: "Yes." This word that confirms your character's experience of the symptoms is not hyperlinked. There is no way to move on in the Twine without selecting the undo arrow that is built into the Harlowe story format. Eventually, to continue the narrative plot, the reader/player must select the final symptom, which includes a hyperlink to a subsequent passage.

While this was a seemingly calculated and effective strategy used by the author to create a sense of regression, other authors used *dead-end* linking in ways that appeared unintentional. *Dead-end* links were coded 21 times in Author 12's story. While some of these links may have been by design to create a particular reader/player experience, the intention of others was less clear. For example, the author devotes many *dead-end* links to passages about their relationship with various family members, including their mother, father, sister and cousin. When the reader/player selects the passage, they are taken to a description of the author's relationship with that person or a description of a significant moment in their shared lives. Two family member passages, the mother and step-brother, are left blank by the author. It is unclear if the blank passages are meant to create meaning around a lack of a relationship with these people, perhaps, or if the author was working under time constraints. Figure 6.4 shows an image of the back end of the Twine structure in the software's interface. The structure of hyperlinks utilized in this Twine reveals that the passage devoted to the mother is actually the only passage that is linked to the larger story structure. The additional family-themed passages include links to one another,

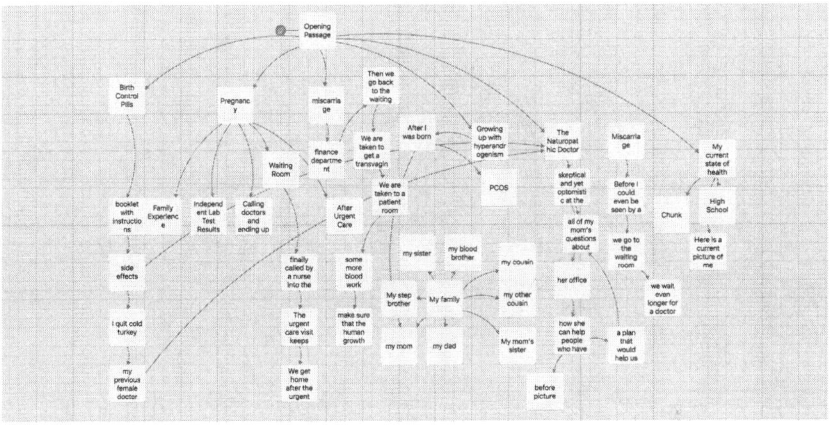


*Figure 6.4* Screenshot of Author 12's Twine Structure.

but not to the larger story structure. The effect this design creates is that none of the family-themed passages, except the mother, can be accessed when the Twine is published. In other words, these passages only truly "exist" in the Twine interface, but not in the published form of the HTML file because there are no hyperlinks that lead to them.

Perhaps this was a mistake by the author. Or, if it was designed purposefully, there is much to be said about the discursive meaning produced by this choice. It creates a salient image of the author seeking, through endless winding paths, familial relationships to no avail. This strategy, or accident, of a passage with no hyperlink access, was found in one other author's story. In the back-end structure of Author 4's Twine, there is a single passage with no hyperlink to the larger story structure. This passage is titled "Normal" and includes no text. The passage cannot be accessed in the published HTML file, but it exists in the interface. This likely was an error made by the author when building their story, however, an inaccessible passage dedicated to the theme of normality produces an added layer of meaning. Normality is just under the surface, in the bones, but the author is unable to reach it.

As depicted in Figure 6.5, *navigational* linking was the dominant linking strategy used by the *Click Me* authors. The reasons why authors relied on *navigational* linking require more research, however, the conceptual impact on the narratives is clear. The dominant use of *navigational* linking, for the *Click Me* narratives, produced a feeling that the reader/player is navigating the story as if it were a space. As Brian Teare argues, in line with the scholarly criticism of narrative medicine's assumptions of the narrative self-outlined in Chapter 1, the illness experience may feel less like a textual story. For Teare, illness is a place. He writes:

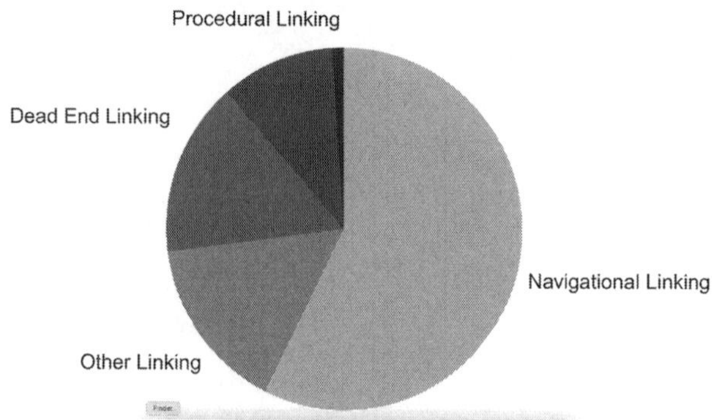


*Figure 6.5* Pie Chart of Linking Strategies Found in Author Narratives.

> The woods of illness were wordless, though they burgeoned with sound, texture, sensation, atmosphere. The somatic experience of illness wasn't narrative: it was place. It was a place my body made out of its chronic disequilibrium, its migraines and nauseas, its gastrointestinal distress and joint pain. There was no story and no map, either. I didn't know how to bring anybody there.
>
> (Teare)

Reimagining the possibilities of space in relation to other material-discursive phenomena is also a core project of feminist new materialism, as outlined in Chapter 3. Karen Barad writes in *Meeting the Universe Halfway* that "With the click of a mouse, space, time, and matter are mutually reconfigured in this cyborg 'trans-action' that transgresses and reworks the boundaries between human and machine, nature and culture, and economic and discursive practices" (223). Barad offers a generative way into looking at how time, space, matter, and discourse become entangled in an affective way. In the case of the *Click Me* narratives, the reader/player is able to tour various narrative moments that are important to the author's illness story. These moments depicted in various passages, through *navigational* linking, become tableaus or vignettes that the reader/player can visit, experience, leave and perhaps return to.

*Navigational* linking, in the stories of the *Click Me* authors, was used in diverging and converging ways to create a sense of spatial touring. Some authors used *navigational* linking to explore past memories as narrative scenes. Author 11, for example, hyperlinked the names of people in their life that are important to their illness journey, including physicians and family members. While this hyperlinking strategy may not initially appear *navigational*, it was coded as such during the analysis of the *Click Me* data. This is because Author 11 designed the narrative to create a sense of spatial navigation. When the reader/player clicks on the name of a person, they are taken to a space dedicated to telling the story of the author's relationship with that character. Rather than advancing the narrative plot in a linear way by detailing a subsequent action, the passage pulls the reader/player back into a memory of the author with this person. Here, the author explores their relationship and the impact this person has on their illness experience. For example, in the opening passage of Author 11's Twine, the reader/player is grappling with the concept of shame. By selecting the hyperlink option [[Dr. 1]], they are brought to a scene of the author at 16 years old sitting in a physician's office learning of their diagnosis for the first time. The narrative then loops back to the opening passage about shame. Selecting [[Sister]], this time, will bring the reader/player to a scene from later in the author's life when they are dealing with infertility amidst their sister's pregnancy. Ultimately, *navigational* linking, in this Twine, centres a narrative that explores emotions around relationships that define moments of an illness, rather than a series of events that play out in order.

Other authors used *navigational* linking for knowledge dissemination. For example, Author 7 designs a Twine that acts as a spatial database of information. The reader/player has hyperlink options to tour the database and learn about the illness of hyperandrogenism, gender identity and the personal experiences of the author. The author writes: "Before I begin sharing my story, it's important for you to understand [[Hyperandrogenism]] is." When the hyperlink is selected, the reader/player is taken to a passage that outlines the definition of the disease, what symptoms accompany it, and the prevalence of its diagnosis in relation to other hormonal disorders. The Twine continues this pedagogical strategy by bringing the reader/player through passages that describe [[polycystic ovary syndrome (PCOS)]], [[What is Gender vs Sex]], and [[hirsutism]]. Through *navigational* linking, this author's Twine acts as both an illness narrative and an interactive tool for the reader/player to learn about various embodiments. In this sense, the Twine is intended to be toured as a definitional database, with added lived experience for context, where there is no "correct" path to take.

While *navigational* linking was used by authors to create a sense of a narrative space, a single spatial location was most commonly described: the waiting room. It might be assumed that other healthcare spaces, such as a physician's office, would be the central, formative space in the story of the illness experience, however, for the *Click Me* authors the waiting room was the dominant thematic space depicted. Several authors used *navigational* linking in their stories to explore the space of a waiting room to depict anxiety around the healthcare encounter as well as feeling intentionally kept in the dark regarding the nature of the illness. For example, Author 12 designed a dynamic Twine narrative that uses *navigational* linking to explore the feeling of being charted through a maze of rooms and left to wait. In the story, the author is experiencing a miscarriage after a period of infertility. The author and their partner rush to visit an urgent care clinic. The author writes:

> we are waiting in the cold waiting room playing soft romantic music from the 80's, which don't sound too romantic now, 6 feet away from each other due to COVID-19 restrictions. My head hangs, I want to cry. I need to cry as I feel like I already know how things will play out. I don't cry, but I feel as though if I could, everything would go away. The physical and emotional pain of everything. I have the feeling that I let everyone down for some reason. I go into the maze when my name is called.

What follows is a series of passages that circle the reader/player through seemingly endless rooms of the clinic, including the finance department to provide health insurance information, a bathroom for a urine sample, and a patient room to complete a lifestyle choices questionnaire. Finally, the author sees a physician that informs the couple that the miscarriage was "complete." The author explains: "There's a knock at the door even before my husband and I can embrace and cry together in privacy." A nurse returns to explain additional tests that are required for the near future. In our closing interview, the author summarizes this experience as being made to feel like they are merely a number in the system.

Salter and Moulthrop further categorize the structure of a Twine passage as either *bifold construction* or *unified construction*. A *bifold construction*, according to the authors, splits the texts of the passage into two distinct parts. The upper section is described as diegetic text that reports the events of the narrative world. The lower section is hypothetical text, consisting of "language still in play" (Salter and Moulthrop 69). This language still in play, according to Salter and Moulthrop, typically includes hypertext options for the reader/player to advance the narrative. A unified construction, in contrast, merges the hypertext and the diegetic text into a single section. As the authors explain, in a unified construction "There are link anchors, but they fit into the diegesis instead of pulling away from it, as is often the case in the bifold scheme" (Salter and Moulthrop 70). Ultimately Salter and Moulthrop outline these two categories to organize the scholarly trajectory of narrative-ness versus game-ness in literary hypertext.

A simplistic analysis would conclude that a "bifold construction accentuates the gamelike qualities of Twine stories, while the unified approach plays to literary interests" however "this distinction can never be absolute" (Salter and Moulthrop 70). Passages in the *Click Me* Twines were coded during data analysis, individually, as either *unified*, *bifold*, or *bi-uni construction*. The latter category captured passages that incorporated aspects of both *bifold* and *unified construction* where hypertexts would be littered throughout the

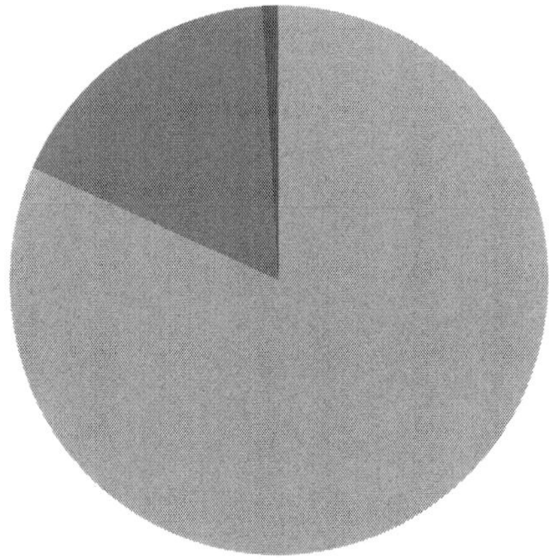


*Figure 6.6* Pie Chart of Passage Construction Strategies Found in Author Narratives.

diegetic upper section, as well as in options for plot advancement in the lower section. As depicted in Figure 6.6, the *Click Me* Twines overwhelmingly included passages of *unified construction*. In line with Salter and Moulthrop's call to resist the urge to filter Twines into a binary of game versus narrative, it may be more valuable to "explore the spaces between those alternatives, refining a new art form as we go" (71). Therefore, no claim will be made regarding the game-ness or narrative-ness of this finding.

Ultimately, while Chapter 5 dissects the ways in which textual discourse creates meaning within and outside of the *Click Me* Twines, this chapter unpacks the additional, affective matter that forms meaning in its own right. The ways in which the authors build their Twines, from the opening passage to whom they decide to share their narratives with, speak to a discursive network that extends beyond the Twine interface and into the world around the authors. This is the intention, I think: if the project is to fortify positive relationships between the identities of the authors and the world, we ultimately need ways to infiltrate the world around us, to impact it, shape it, and change the way it interacts with our sense of identities and our physical bodies. The *Click Me* authors, I found, were engaged in these ideas in ways I did not expect, but were notably powerful.

## Mapping the Illness Narrative

The most compelling finding of the *Click Me* research was how the authors spoke about the therapeutic potential of using literary hypertext technology to write illness narratives. Authors, in different ways, explored the concept of using the digital features of Twine to visually map out their experiences, and manually organize them by hyperlinking passages, to find a structure that the author felt was best suited for personal reflection. Authors used language such as "constructing an experiential chart," a "map," a "planner," a "puzzle" or a "web," to convey this phenomenon. Collectively, authors described how the ability to physically and spatially organize their illness narrative into passages, that can be linked in various ways and situated in a linear/nonlinear path, created a unique and effective resource for the author to design an individualized therapeutic resource for reflecting on experience. Author 1 explains:

> I think it made me think more about like how things like fit in together and how certain parts of like my experience might be related…that was really interesting using like, the flow chart style kind of in that way.

Similarly, Author 16 notes: "It was almost like a choose-your-own-adventure, except in this way, it was just more so all of the decisions that I was creating, was still leading to the end result, which was very relatable to my life." This shared sentiment of the therapeutic value of mapping the illness narrative through hypertext and passages was discussed by authors in four different ways: a belief that writing with Twine mirrors the human thought process, matches the experience of an illness diagnosis, conveys the feeling of a negative mental health circuit, and facilitates personal discoveries through the practice of hyperlinking.

Some authors made claims that the rhizomatic structure of Twine "mirrored" how they perceived the brain engages in thought process, and therefore the software is well suited to build personal narratives. Author 4 describes their belief that mapping out their illness narrative in Twine, through branching hypertexts, "mirrors the way that we think." The author explains:

> Sometimes your memories will trigger other, other things that have happened, you know? And so by, by planning it out this way, I was able to kind of channel some of that, like, yeah, there was this event, oh, and then and then this happened, or these are the kinds of things that were going through my mind. And I think it actually better captures how we think in general.

In contrast, Author 1 discussed how they believed their "brain worked" in a more linear fashion where it felt more authentic to them to design a forward path, rather than multiple paths. The author explains:

> I think the platform still like worked really well for that [linear storytelling] and I liked that it was like, there was like a heading, and you could

> travel between like different… because it was kind of broken up into little topics, I guess. And I used like one hyperlink to like jump forward reading about another part.

Author 1 explained that, although Twine may be traditionally used to create nonlinear narratives, building a forward path with thematic passages still had a therapeutic impact. Rather than reinforce any claims about inherent processes of the brain, what is significant, here, is a belief system that authors cultivate around how literary hypertext facilitates their writing effectively. They are arguing that the technology, in different ways, offers a useful method to brainstorm their thoughts, organize their narrative structure and build their stories. This may be through utilizing branching narrative paths or creating a linear story with thematic passages.

Authors made claims about how the Twine software cultivated emotional breakthroughs via the hyperlink feature. Author 5 described how they wrote about different life experiences in multiple passages. Initially, they believed that these anecdotes were emotionally distinct moments. The author incidentally chose the same thematic word to be a hyperlink in each passage. It was when the author saw two passages physically link to each other in the Twine interface, via the use of the same hyperlink thematic word that they recognized the two experiences as emotionally bound. The author explained: "there was a point where I made it more like a bulk text, but I was able to actually break it down. And then like, see the links between them." This author is describing a concept of a physical link in the software cultivating a cognitive link that becomes important to the therapeutic process. This is compelling insight because it speaks to how Twine might facilitate therapeutic reflection through digital features, rather than the act of writing an illness narrative alone.

Authors shared a common belief, reflected on in closing interviews, that the rhizomatic capabilities of literary hypertext embody the feeling of an illness diagnosis. Author 12 discussed their belief that writing in Twine matches the feeling one experiences when one receives an illness diagnosis. They explain:

> I think in like in the sense of writing a nonlinear story where I can just kind of go all over the place with kind of the narrative and what I wanted to get across. I think that's really helpful. Because with hyperandrogenism and PCOS–these conditions just kind of make your brain just kind of scattered all over the place. So it is kind of nice to know that I don't have to start at the beginning that I can go to different places, and be like, 'oh, yeah, that is connected. That does make sense'.

Author 4 discussed similar insight, explaining that in the aftermath of an illness diagnosis, a patient is forced to consider an influx of questions and anxieties: "You're, you're going through so much, and you're thinking about so much and like, what are the implications? What is the [sic] diagnosis mean? How do I have to change my lifestyle?" Akin to Arthur Frank's argument that illness disrupts this planned destination of our life, illness diagnoses mushrooms our projection of a linear life path into a web of endless possibilities, or in other words, the unknown. For these authors, the inherent structure of Twine helped them capture this feeling.

Ultimately, the belief systems that emerged for authors from mapping their illness narratives in Twine can be summarized by the astute reflection of Author 7 who refers to this phenomenon as the intersectional "web of our identity." The author notes:

> I think specifically in using Twine where you can link everything I think it really just talked to like the web of our identity and how everything kind of comes together. Versus if it was, you know, making a video or writing a story, I think it just gives more space to kind of link and ties different parts of like who I am together.

For this author, and others, the web of identity is rooted in experiences of intersectionality. Author 7 explains how writing their illness narrative in Twine "highlighted for me my intersectionality of like, this is one piece." They go on to explain that their illness, along with their gender and many other elements of who they are, are single pieces of their experience that all intersect to create their identity. The author reflects:

> I think that to me, [Twine] kind of just gave space, I think for like, kind of some of the intersectionality of the experience and as much as it's like, all one part of identity, it is different aspects of it.

The digital features of Twine, in this sense, both deconstructed and reconstructed this identity web in ways that allowed some authors to gain a more comprehensive understanding and therapeutic reflection of their illness experience.

**Twine, Resistance and Capacity**

As of the time this book was written, Chris Klimas hosts a Patreon account to fund periodic software releases related to the Twine project where he notes that he maintains a full-time job in addition to his contribution to Twine. Patreon is a platform that facilitates membership funding for creative projects, in exchange for access to exclusive content, community and insight. Alternatively, Twine suggests supporting the maintenance of its infrastructure through donations to The Interactive Technology Foundation, a nonprofit organization that provides support for the interactive fiction community. In keeping with Twine's spirit of collective contribution, the site encourages nonfinancial support such as drafting answers to user questions, contributing to the official Cookbook, fixing software bugs, or translating the user interface into other languages.

According to the GitHub source code, Twine 2 was written using various programming languages including HTML5 and JavaScript. The Twine software is open-source and, as of the time this book was written, is maintained by a collective of individuals on several different repositories through GitHub and other development platforms. GitHub, and its culture of supporting collaborative version control of, typically, open-source projects speaks to Twine's identity as an inclusive space of collective contribution and creation. As Salter and Moulthrop argue, Twine can stand as an equalizer in a classroom where students hold differing experiences with programming, technology and digital literacy because, at its core, the software is a tool to make the personal political. Salter and Moulthrop argue, "Twine is a tool for resisting the dominant interactive storytelling of our times and, as such, tends to be a tool for chronicling resistance and struggle" (Salter and Moulthrop 2).

This praise is a lot to live up to, I think. I was compelled in this research to highlight how literary hypertext embodied this vehicle for accessible personalized resistance. I found it did, in many ways. Though, I found moments where courage did not align with conviction, as with any grand statements of liberatory accessibility. These moments harken back to Couser's point about certain illnesses or disabilities that can limit how a person is able to write or publish their story. Outlined in Chapter 1, Couser was referring to more traditional writing and publishing practices in relation to partnerships such as assisting authors, transcribers, translators, ghostwriters and the kinds of ethical issues that can emerge. However, this appears to be true in some ways for Twine as well. Despite Twine championing accessible, anti-establishment game development, it is still inaccessible in many ways for those living with particular illnesses or disabilities. For example, Twine stories may be compatible with screen readers, but this feature is contingent on intentional technical design and story format choices made by the author. It is vital to have experience incorporating sets of roles and attributes that define ways to make web content more accessible to people with disabilities.

Twine today is multifaceted; it is haunted by the aftermath of Gamergate and increased misogyny in the gaming community, the COVID-19 pandemic and disruptions to the supply chain, the sky-rocketing cost of living due to inflation, global climate change-induced natural disasters, and increased risk of the loss of human rights. What I learned from the *Click Me* authors in this study was that you can have the most technologically accessible tool to create narratives aimed at elevating emotional well-being, however, capacity, in all its forms including physical, mental, financial, and temporal, to sit down and learn a new technology is a privilege. In addition to outlining the sociohistorical legacy of Twine as a tool of resistance for those pushed to the margins of game development, it is important in this book to note the real-life ways in which power relations monopolize capacity.

## Therapeutic Value of Literary Hypertext Illness Narratives

In closing interviews, the *Click Me* authors were asked to describe their feelings towards their body, identity, or ideas about where they fit in the world after writing about their illness. This question included further prompts that aimed to identify if authors believed writing their literary hypertext illness narrative was an impactful experience, in various ways. Overwhelmingly, authors reiterated the same belief: that writing a single illness narrative, in any format, cannot (and is not intended to) "cure" or "fix" the self. After writing a single Twine narrative, one will not suddenly develop an encompassing positive body image or resolve past illness trauma. This finding is aligned with the second-wave scholars of hypertext, emerging in the 2000s, who cautioned against overenthusiastic declarations of literary hypertext's emancipatory capabilities.

Scholars such as Ensslin, Pope, Miall and Mangen argue that the liberatory value of literary hypertext can be cultivated through careful and strategic adoption of immersive, adaptable and user-friendly practices (Ensslin and Skains 8). At the core, however, is the centring of co-creation modalities. Second-wave hypertext scholars conclude that the transformative potential of the medium is found through collaborative methods that empower the reader's contribution to the text's creation and actively deconstruct binaries between the author and the reader/player. In the *Click Me* research, there are no reader/players. Or, alternatively, I as the researcher have become the reader, as well as the *Click Me* authors who have read each other's stories. This project, though, resists a stark dichotomy of author/reader by eliminating the subject position of reader all together. The focus is on the author and the experience of writing the narrative, which is a method of challenging subject positions.

The consensus from the *Click Me* authors was that engaging in writing a literary hypertext illness narrative was impactful and beneficial because it facilitated reflection on past experiences. This process of reflection, for authors, ultimately led to new vantage points to better understand emotions, the establishment of a connection to the self, and validation of experiences of injustice. Authors agreed that their writing of a literary hypertext illness narrative did not produce a purely transformative, curative outcome. What the authors noted was an impactful opportunity to reflect on past experiences and gain a new, productive perspective. For example, Author 16 explains:

> I don't want to say that there was like this crazy positive impact after writing it, but I do think it kind of, for me, it was more so like a looking back as to like, where I was first where I am now.

The author goes on to explain their personal growth in overcoming a sense of hopelessness to ultimately embrace "self-love" regardless of what their body looks like. This transformation took place before the author wrote their narrative, however, the writing process allowed them to reflect on it.

Author 1 described using the writing process as a tool of reflection through a method of juxtaposing positive and negative experiences. They explain:

> I think that going through the writing process allowed me to...think about all of the negative interactions I'd had and like, kind of add those up. And then all of the positive interactions I'd had and like compare them to each other.

This sentiment was mirrored in the answer of another author who expressed uncertainty about whether any single experience can completely change one's self-perception. This author explained that the writing process allowed them to bring past illness experiences to the forefront of their attention, which they typically resist. Finding this time to centre and reflect on their illness experience, for this author, emboldened them to connect with the healthcare system again. The author explains that they made an appointment with their physician for the following day. Further, they shared that deciding to join the study prompted them to contact their family doctor and seek a specialist for hyperandrogenism. For this author, reflecting on their experience of illness through writing emboldened them to revisit a treatment plan in the normative healthcare system.

There was a recurring theme, in closing interviews, of the writing process allowing for a novel vantage point to reflect on the illness experience from a removed space. Author 10, for example, shared that it took them a long time to write their narrative. They recall putting the module off because it felt "triggering'" and "overwhelming" to dig up the emotional experiences they have had over the past several years. It was "serendipitous," according to the author, that I eventually sent them a follow-up email, inquiring if they were still interested in participating in the *Click Me* study because they finally felt ready to write. The author explained: "so that weekend like I took a whole Sunday and I just sat with everything that whole Sunday, it was a very, very quiet day. And I just wrote down everything." Ultimately, the author notes,

> it felt really good to actually just write it out and get it out. And yeah, kind of put it into perspective. It was like me not being part of it anymore, but kind of being out of it and looking at it from out here.

Author 9 shared a similar sentiment, describing the convention of writing something down that you want to remember. They explained that "you can't really shrug something off because it's already written. It's there, it's there for the world to see." In writing, the hardship of the experience becomes immortalized, and this allowed them to recognize their courage in navigating the pain. Ultimately, the author believes the writing process to be different from sharing their experience in person. In the past, when living in a different country, the author felt unsafe sharing their experience of infertility with others. The author explains:

> The thing that I'm trying to avoid is people, like, people…pitying me because I'm going through that stuff. So when I was writing, I was like, no one's gonna know, or no one's gonna judge me or no one's gonna feel bad for me or feel sorry for me… it relieved me of the burden that I've been carrying for years.

Ultimately, the author concludes that while sharing their experiences is important to them, it is difficult to talk about the past and easier to write about.

The *Click Me* authors described that the writing process helped them understand themselves better. This outcome was discussed by authors in different ways including finding a resolution for past emotions or discovering a sense of identity. Author 11 shared that they wrote about a negative emotional reaction they had when they heard the news that their sister was pregnant. Writing about this time helped the author process a sense of shame around infertility. The author explained:

> I'm realizing that it was the shame that was actually causing that, like, the fact that I've been working so hard and couldn't get something that's so easy for other people. I think it gave me a better understanding of the emotions attached to it.

This reflective process had real-world impacts on the life of the author. They discussed: "That was a really big moment because she actually just found out she's pregnant again. We reacted much differently this time. And we've talked about that." This author was able to use the writing process as a way to understand their responses better to ultimately address the relationships in their life.

Author 12 discussed a similar reckoning with the self in relation to gender embodiment through writing. They describe:

> before the study, I just, I have just a lot of confusion and a lot of just anger towards my body…But now it was more of like, just trying to more identify who, who I really am. And trying to figure out, you know, how, how I'm in between two different worlds, or multiple worlds, if that makes sense. And then by being kind of processing this, and writing things down. I came to a place where I was like, at the end of the day, it's just, I'm just me. I'm just myself.

The author comes to the conclusion that despite the feeling of existing between multiple worlds, they can remain grounded in themselves. It is poetic to think about the relationship between Twine and the self as inverse. In the software, the author starts at a central passage and branches outward into multiple paths. But for this author, their "multitude of worlds" was honed in through their writing experience to a central point of self.

One of the main outcomes discussed by the *Click Me* authors in the closing interviews was that writing their illness narratives in literary hypertext facilitated a sense of validation of the injustice they experienced. While some authors believed they were not able to feel validation in the moment, seeing their experience written out in the interface legitimized for them that what they experienced was, in fact, unjust. For example, Author 10 reflected on their experience with a "fatphobic" physician who coldly advised the author to lose weight without acknowledging the myriad of factors contributing to their embodied experience. The author wrote about wanting to "spit in his face" at that moment but ultimately did nothing. Although the author could not stand up to this act of perceived discrimination at the time, writing about the experience affirmed, for the author, that they experienced injustice.

This sense of not only contending with the injustice of the past but also actively imagining a new future world is the bones of feminist new materialism. I am reminded of the concepts of *situated feminisms* and *speculative fabulation*, both of which were coded in the analysis of the data of the *Click Me* Twines. These are feminist new materialism concepts, described by Truman as mirrored energy. Situated feminisms is concerned with an ethical inhabitation that recognizes the self as deeply intertwined with a network of matter, both human and nonhuman. This situated knowledge, according to Truman, is a feminist new materialist "project towards a different world." This different world is found through speculative fabulation or imagining how the world can be. Truman brings in the theories of Elizabeth Grosz in her 2004 book *The Nick of Time: Politics, Evolution, and the Untimely*, to fortify "how political and cultural struggles focus on a both reconfiguring

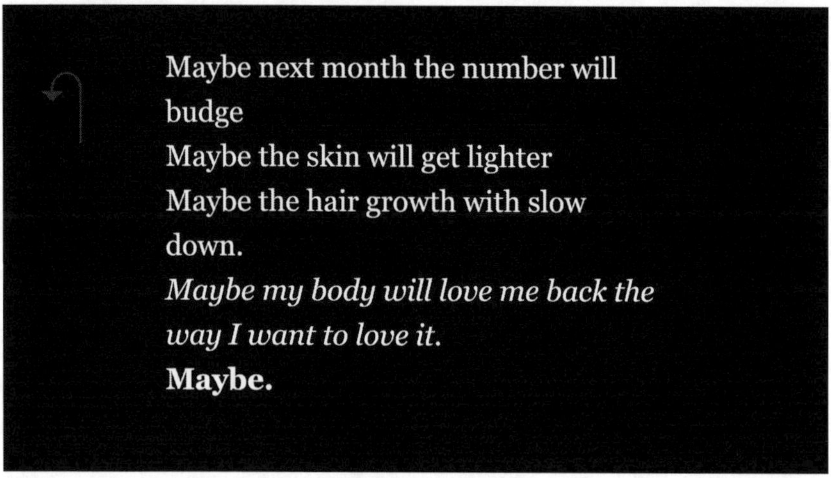


*Figure 6.7* Screenshot of Author 16's Twine Story.

the past to rectify injustices" as well as a process of limitless, ongoing world-building by imagining what the future can be and past could have been (7). This feminist new materialist exercise emerged in the narratives of the *Click Me* research. Authors wrote about past injustices and how the material realities of prejudice and pathology come to be in their lives. What was less stark, but budding, in these narratives was a feminist imagining of a more just world. For example, speculative fabulation is embodied in the final passage of Author 16's narrative as shown in Figure 6.7. It is the final two lines, set apart from the rest of the text by different styling, where a future world is imagined: maybe.

### Literary Hypertext Illness Narratives as a Teaching Tool

The previous section details how the *Click Me* authors reiterated a common belief that writing an illness narrative in literary hypertext does not have a holistic, curative effect on the self but can offer a valuable opportunity to reflect on past experiences. Authors, however, also came to an additional conclusion. This additional conclusion, I believe, truly pushes this project beyond the scope of individualized therapeutic solutions to implicate power relations at play within institutional structures. Ultimately, I began this research by pulling illness narratives as a method out of narrative medicine as a practice (as outlined in Chapter 1). However, the *Click Me* authors seem to refortify this connection by calling for an integration of patient narratives in clinical practice, research, and education. This is the basis of a narrative medicine approach and akin to Martinez and Fleck-Henderson's notion of health liberation. The *Click Me* authors explained that the distress that accompanies hyperandrogenism is rooted in the way the disease is taken up culturally. Therefore, for literary hypertext illness narratives about hyperandrogenism to cultivate true therapeutic value, they should be a tool, not only for the author to reflect on the experience but also for the wider community to read and learn about the experience of hyperandrogenism.

Authors spoke about the desire to share illness narratives in various ways, including formally in a healthcare education setting or informally through social media platforms such as TikTok. Author 11 explains: "I thought about sharing my, my Twine, like somewhere. I don't know where." The author goes on to explain that they wanted to share their story in a place that would cultivate awareness of the experience of hyperandrogenism amongst people in their community. They note: "I don't think like even people…understand like, like the teacher that told me like, oh, that it's fake. Or the doctor that only wanted to deal with my skin tags and nothing else." Author 10 dives deeper into this belief by acknowledging that literary hypertext illness narratives would be a beneficial method in a formal therapy session. The benefit of this tool, according to the author, would be amplified by its accessibility to healthcare professionals who deal with hyperandrogenism so they can gain an understanding of the lived experience of the disease. The author astutely notes:

> it would be even cooler if it [Twine illness narratives] was actually like a medical tool as well, right? Like, if doctors and healthcare providers could also be on board that it's not just a therapy thing…but it's also like a very real thing that needs…very real care that needs to happen, right? Like, either medicine needs to be prescribed or things need to happen and change.

This sentiment was mirrored by other authors as well. Author 3, for example, explained that they felt that for a PCOS patient, there were institutionalized issues in the healthcare system that acted as a barrier to humanized treatment. The author wonders if they had access to a "collection of, like, people's stories like this" if they would be able to map a pattern that points to the reasons that underpin systemic injustice in the healthcare system.

In the end, I believe the *Click Me* authors have convinced me. They shared highly personal stories of living with a *sick* identity in a world that is incongruent with *sickness*. They also built narratives of trauma that outline the harm they have experienced from contact with the normative healthcare system. While my initial reaction was to perhaps throw the baby out with the normative healthcare system and build new systems of access, I am convinced, now, that there is space to grow within. By calling for the inclusion of their stories in clinical practice, research and education, the *Click Me* authors echo the principles of narrative medicine and health liberation. This call reveals that the distress associated with hyperandrogenism is deeply intertwined with cultural perceptions and systemic issues within healthcare and this is where the work needs to start.

## Works Cited

Barad, Karen. *Meeting the Universe Halfway: Quantum Physics and the Entanglement of Matter and Meaning*. Duke University Press, 2007.

Ensslin, Astrid, and Lyle Skains. "Hypertext: Storyspace to Twine." *The Bloomsbury Handbook of Electronic Literature*, edited by Joseph Tabbi, Bloomsbury Publishing, 2017, pp. 295–310.

Frank, Arthur W. *The Wounded Storyteller: Body, Illness, and Ethics*, 2nd ed. The University of Chicago Press, 2013.

Grosz, Elizabeth. *The Nick of Time: Politics, Evolution, and the Untimely*. Routledge, 2020.

Hayles, N. Katherine. "Print is Flat, Code is Deep: The Importance of Media-Specific Analysis." *Poetics Today*, vol. 25, no. 1, 2004, pp. 67–90.

Mangen, Anne and Adriaan van der Weel. "Why Don't We Read Hypertext Novels?" *Convergence*, vol. 23, no. 2, 2017, pp. 166–181.

Miall, David and Teresa Dobson. "Reading Hypertext and the Experience of Literature." *Journal of Digital Information*, vol. 2, no. 1, 2001. Online Journal.

Pope, James. "A Future for Hypertext Fiction." *Convergence*, vol. 12, no. 4, 2006, pp. 447–465.

Richardson, Rick T., et al. "Color and Contrast in E-Learning Design: A Review of the Literature and Recommendations for Instructional Designers and Web Developers." *MERLOT Journal of Online Learning and Teaching*, vol. 10, no. 4, 2014, pp. 657–670.

Salter, Anastasia, and Stuart Moulthrop. *Twining*. Amherst College Press, 2021.

Teare, Brian. "Neither Chaos Nor Quest: Toward a Nonnarrative Medicine." *The Boston Review*, 3 February 2022, https://www.bostonreview.net/articles/neither-chaos-nor-quest-toward-a-nonnarrative-medicine/#:~:text=Narrative%20medicine%20claims%20to%20champion,what%20is%20wrong%20with%20them. Accessed 5 Dec. 2022.

Truman, Sarah E. "Feminist New Materialisms." *SAGE Research Methods*, 2020.

*Twine Cookbook*. Twinery.org, 2021, https://twinery.org/cookbook/

# 7 The Future of Digital Illness Narratives

## Why Hyperandrogenism? Why Now?

Across a countless number of jurisdictions we have seen a surge in what has been dubbed "anti-trans laws." In 2024, there were an unprecedented 88 bills introduced at the federal level in the United States that intersect with healthcare, student athletics, the military, incarceration, and education (Trans Legislation Tracker). As of early 2025, three Canadian provinces have introduced laws and policies that many argue restrict transgender rights—most severely, in this author's home province of Alberta. A trio of bills—the *Education Amendment Act* (Bill 27), the *Health Statutes Amendment Act* (Bill 26), and the *Fairness and Safety in Sport Act* (Bill 29)—have been introduced. These emerging "anti-trans laws" in Alberta, which have been publicly condemned by Amnesty International (Amnesty International Canada), telegraph a growing shadow over the state of rights for people living with hyperandrogenism worldwide. The fight for transgender rights and the rights of those with hyperandrogenism are interconnected under the shared goal of bodily autonomy. While these laws explicitly target transgender people, the political issues surrounding transgender identities and hyperandrogenism are deeply intertwined.

Globally, the emergence of these "anti-trans laws" are wholly ambiguous regarding if hyperandrogenism is carved in or out of scope. For example, Arizona Senate Bill 1138 bans physicians from providing gender reassignment surgery to minors. However, the Bill states that a physician may offer to minors:

> Services provided when a physician has otherwise diagnosed a disorder of sexual development and has determined through genetic or biochemical testing that the individual does not have normal sex chromosome structure, sex steroid hormone production, or sex steroid hormone action.
>
> (Arizona State Legislature)

DOI: 10.4324/9781003646921-7

In contrast, while hyperandrogenism has been absent in the public discourse surrounding Alberta's Bill 26, this author would argue that the legislation is unclear. Bill 26 prohibits regulated health professionals from prescribing hormone replacement therapies including puberty blockers to minors for the treatment of "gender dysphoria" or "gender incongruence" (Legislative Assembly of Alberta, *the Health Statutes Amendment Act*) where the latter is defined as "a marked and persistent incongruence between a person's gender identity and that person's sex assigned at birth" (Legislative Assembly of Alberta, *Health Professions Act*). Where can we plot the affects of expression, materially, bodily changes, distress, prescriptions drugs, modifications and more that emerge alongside the hyperandrogenous experience on the map of "persistent incongruence"? Where does hyperandrogenism live here?

Second, there is a real threat that these "anti-trans laws" will create a barrier for people with hyperandrogenism to learn about themselves and understand that there are others like them in the world. Alberta's Bill 27, for example, requires parental notification and consent before students engage in learning about "gender identity, sexual orientation, or human sexuality" (Legislative Assembly of Alberta, *the Education Amendment Act*). Further, it mandates that educational resources focused on these topics be approved by the Minister of Education unless used for religious instruction. Where do the experiences of hyperandrogenism fit into the category of "gender identity"? There is a stark farcical impact in co-opting language of the political left but presenting it void of the nuance this language embodies.

Third, to revisit the issue of hyperandrogenism in sport, many of these "anti-trans laws" may work to further restrict participation in sports for adults and youth with hyperandrogenism. Alberta's Bill 29 will require organizations subject to the Act to create athlete eligibility policies. The Act refrains from explicit reference to women or gender, however, the provincial government has publicly contextualized the Act as intended to ensure "women and girls have the opportunity to compete in biological female-only divisions" (Government of Alberta, *Ensuring Fairness and Safety in Sport*). This will leave individual agencies responsible for creating eligibility requirements for participation. I ask here again: where will athletes with hyperandrogenism be considered, or not considered, within this framework of inclusion and exclusion in sport?

I want to, here, return to the story of Caster Semenya. Her treatment in public discourse, and by athletic governing bodies, is situated as an antecedent to this book. Semenya's story is presented in the Twine module used by the *Click Me* authors, where they engage with public discourse, the scrutiny of the IAAF, and Semenya's own reflections on her experiences of dehumanization. Semenya's story has become one of a handful of cases plucked from the ether and chosen to wholly represent a global, multifaceted issue surrounding the dynamics of differing bodies in sport. These athletes—Semenya included—who do not present neatly within a sex-based category have ignited a frenzy of anxieties that lay bare the white underbelly of our culture's racist, sexist, transphobic and homophobic affinities.

The regulation of gender identity and expression is metastasizing across the globe, and these political mandates that target the most vulnerable and small populations of our communities reflect a more insidious/targeted/coordinated push to legislate the restriction of bodily autonomy for particular abject bodies. In the end, even if these "anti-trans laws," and the aligned sociopolitical war on transgender people, did not intersect with hyperandrogenous experience, the loss of liberty for one is a loss of freedom for all.

Ultimately, Semenya's story teaches us that we are a culture that sees ourselves as nourishing diversity but, in the final reckoning, our fear tends to prevail and the abnormal bodies that make rich our communities are pushed to the margins. In a 2023 op-ed for the *New York Times*, Semenya notes:

> No one suggested Michael Phelps's dominance in the pool was unfair and he should have to take medication to ensure that he produced just as much lactic acid as his competitors or have surgery to fix his hypermobile joints. The swimmer Katie Ledecky was never accused of being a man because she smashed multiple world records and her ever-improving times in several events would qualify her for the men's Olympic trials. But they said such things about me because I represented something that was seen as abnormal.

This abnormality for Semenya, for the *Click Me* authors, for me, and perhaps even for you, reader, is what makes us dangerous. I wonder, though, if the project of re-narrating our lives, and our world, turns the danger into power? That is, after all, the hope of the *Click Me* research and the true question at the heart of this book: how do we re-narrate danger as power?

When I started this research many years ago, fuelled by, admittedly, personal negative experiences in the normative healthcare system, I had envisioned hypertext illness narratives as a sort of small-scale, individual whistleblowing mechanism to expose and condemn systemic responses to hyperandrogenism. What was unexpected was that the whistleblowing from the *Click Me* authors turned out to be a plea for community. To evoke the branching rhizome, the ultimate final act for the *Click Me* authors was not to expose the root of the system, but to plant seeds of change. They want to see others like themselves treated with dignity in the healthcare system. Even more, they want individuals with experiences of hyperandrogenism to be clinicians in the healthcare system—to be nurses, physicians, psychologists and insurance providers. They want, ultimately, to mend the system from within. Perhaps investing in novel, innovative approaches to therapy, including hypertext illness narratives, is a step to meet the *Click Me* authors' call to action. But, as the authors astutely note, one action—or one new therapy method—will not overhaul a lifetime of being made to feel abnormal in your skin. The next question is: how do we work together to create deep systemic change—socially within our families and cultures, institutionally in our medical system, athletic programs and schools, and most critically, within ourselves? I have a deep, optimistic hope that this is work yet to come.

In this final chapter, we will revisit the key arguments presented throughout this book. In the following section you will find an overview of the limitations and barriers of the research at the heart of this book. Next, a detailed summary of the main findings in relation to the *Click Me* research question is presented. Then we will move through a discussion of the main contributions of this book, including application beyond the academic literature. As discussed throughout this book, the *Click Me* Twine illness narratives are intended to be accessible for individuals to write in isolation. This research is meant to stand as one response to illness that may be taken outside, within or alongside the normative healthcare system, including formal psychological therapy. The nuances of mediating this application will be detailed below. Finally, recommendations for future research will be discussed in relation to emerging technologies. Here, we will turn to look to the future of literary hypertext and illness narratives as a whole and ask the following question: what's next?

## Limitations, Oversights and Barriers

The research at the heart of this book was bound by particular restrictions, errors and oversights. I believe it is important to open this final chapter by laying these realities out on the figurative lawn for our neighbours to gawk at—if only to help the next person to design a research plan that learns from my mistakes. The limitations of this project include the legacy of previous research, the participant pool and world events. There is no foundational research that could be drawn on in this project related to literary hypertext illness narratives and marginalized identities. This was a barrier to the development of integral parts of the book, including the work that was conducted around a literature review and setting the tone for an effective methodology. Many sections of this book, because it is interdisciplinary, required a Frankenstein approach to design that pulled pieces of different frameworks and meshed them together. While in some areas this became an advantage because it facilitates a curated and individualized approach to the development of the research, it was a limitation to the literature review. It would have been beneficial to have a set of previous studies and articles more closely related to this topic to build on.

The demographic makeup of the *Click Me* participants was generally diverse. I believe there was important representation among individuals who embodied various identities related to race, ability, health, gender, body size and sexuality. Representation lacked, or failed to be measured, in class and age. There was no reporting of socioeconomic class identity in the screening interview of the *Click Me* project. This was an intentional decision. There was ample consideration of how to include a self-reported question in the interview regarding class, but the nuances of this were complex. Class identity is a contentious space between and outside of education, income, employment status, residence, life history, etc. The risk of getting this identity marker wrong outweighed the benefit of including this data in the book. Age was a question included in the screening interviews and this data revealed that *Click Me* participants were relatively young (all authors were in their 20s or 30s). There is more to be analyzed in the recruitment methods of this project that appears to have been exclusionary to older individuals. This may be due to the online recruitment methods and the online nature of the *Click Me* study. Additional factors may be contributing as well including understanding who is more inclined to be seeking alternative ways to respond to hyperandrogenism and why.

Many would consider the participant pool as an evident limitation of this study. There were ten authors who completed the *Click Me* module and submitted their narratives in this research. This is a limited number of participants which prevents the research from being able to make any sort of broad claims about the findings. The findings of this book are relevant to the nuanced and detailed experiences of a small number of people. However, there are benefits to the pool size as well. Because of the embodied and experiential nature of this research, I was able to produce a mass amount of data from a small number of participants. I spent time with each author, listened to their story and shared my own. They gave hours of their life as well. This sort of deep reciprocal bond is rare in research conducted on large participant pools and I feel lucky I was able to hold this space in this project.

The *Click Me* research began at the start of the COVID-19 pandemic, which led to unexpected disruptions in the design of this project. I was debating conducting the participant research as an in-person workshop, but this idea was quickly discarded after March 2020. To protect authors, adhere to local and national guidelines, and to accommodate geographical location, the *Click Me* study was designed to take place entirely online. The pandemic mandating the online nature of the research, in fact, was less of a limitation to this work than the mental and emotional toll isolation inflicted on authors and myself. As discussed in previous chapters of this book, technology can be unmatched in its gift of access, however, this access can only go so far.

It does not respond to the capacity required to sit down and learn a new software and spend time reflecting on emotional experiences.

**Final Discoveries and Insights**

This book began (and will end) with the central theme of the impact of narrative: how sharing our stories can catalyze both personal therapeutic and larger systemic change. Chapter 1 explores the fundamental medium of illness narrative and traces its social and scholarly interpretations across various spaces. We began with the sentiments of Arthur Frank's *The Wounded Storyteller* where he argues that the experience of major illness can destabilize the linear, progressive narrative path we construct about our lives. This path is predicated on the assumption of health. Receiving an unexpected diagnosis acts as an intervention into this path and the trajectory we envisioned for our *selves* and, subsequently, our lives, begins to unravel. In its place—to abuse the tree metaphor—this path becomes a dense forest with no clear throughline. Our life becomes uncertain and populated with symptoms, clinic waiting rooms and foreign diagnoses. This is where we adopt the *sick* identity—a new label that plunges some of us into a relationship with the normative medical institution. In patient–clinician encounters, we surrender our life story to the system, and in turn, the system rewrites our narrative in a language that is no longer accessible to us. Frank, Couser and other scholars of illness narrative argue that taking ownership of our life stories is the ultimate act of reclaiming agency for the *sick* identity.

While the literature on illness narratives establishes its impact as an effective therapeutic method, there are valid and deeply critical barriers to access for marginalized authors that require attention–within, outside and alongside the academy. Chapter 1 reflects on criticisms regarding the limited access to illness narratives by contrasting it with the distinct medium of literary hypertext. Because this generally accessible medium is revolutionizing access to game design and storytelling for marginalized communities, the intention of this book has been to carve, or link, a path for illness narratives through hypertext.

Chapter 2 of this book is a grappling with the impacts, aftermaths and affects of the ways in which hyperandrogenism is pathologized in our culture. We introduce, here, the controversial history of "sex verification" testing in global sports and the continued, relentless subjugation these practices inflict on raced bodies. This chapter then meanders through the theoretical literature on discourse, norms, and "intersex" bodies in the linguistic turn, drawing from Georges Canguilhem's work on the historical construction of normativity and pathologization, Judith Butler and Michel Foucault's expansions on these foundational ideas, and an analysis of compulsory able-bodiedness and heteronormativity.

Chapter 3 introduces this project's theoretical framework of feminist new materialism. It asks what the role of matter is in a poststructuralist research project that intersects with narrative discourse, technology, hyperlinks and body hair. Ultimately, it wonders how we can amplify the narratives of the *Click Me* authors in ways that go beyond a thematic analysis of their words to include a dynamic look at the digital-material relational words generated in the affects of their lives, stories, abnormal bodies, etc. Similarly, this chapter argues in favour of the researcher implicating themselves in their research, in ways that pay attention to the affective nature of research. This call, I found, was one of the most meaningful kinship-producing aspects of the *Click Me* research.

Hypertext, as both a scholarly field of study and a social movement, is then introduced. By looking at the broader topic of electronic literature, this chapter navigates through the emergence of hypertext in the 1960s and the evolution of the technology alongside its functionality. As Twine emerges as a key actor in the discourse surrounding hypertext as a democratizing tool for game development, there has also been a cultural backlash against efforts for inclusivity in the game industry exemplified by movements like #GamerGate. What we learned, in the context of the *Click Me* project, is that digital mediation is a beast by design. To live in our time is to know this beast. Once content is released into the online space for consumption and commentary, it is free to live and die by the public's will, beyond the control of the author. While this mediation can be a catalyst for community-building, it also carries inherent risks. The Twines created by *Click Me* authors do not exist in the public online space due to these risks. Yet, what is overlooked, or absent, in what this decision represents, has been at the forefront of my mind. Who holds the power in digital mediation? Is it the power of the people or the masses that can propel a video to viral territory, for example? Or is it the power inherent in corporations that own digital platforms and design algorithms that dictate the content we consume? See, this question becomes significant in therapeutic digital storytelling, where community-building holds therapeutic value. Perhaps the next step for digital illness narratives would be an investment into creating safe and accessible online spaces for therapeutic narrative sharing in a digitally mediated world. This is a profoundly important project that ultimately needs collective action.

In Chapter 4, I detail a guide for you to build your own hypertext module and this module serves a dual purpose. While its main objective is to facilitate the hypertext illness narrative writing process through a politicized narrative therapy framework, it also acts as a pedagogical tool to teach reader/players the rhizomatic and technical aspects of Twine development. My intention is for this guide to serve individuals and practitioners with little to no knowledge of literary hypertext and to provide an example of how to build a narrative therapy-informed module for facilitating illness narrative writing. Modules informed by this chapter can guide students, patients, healthcare providers and even ourselves.

The module in action is unpacked in Chapters 5 and 6 where narrative themes of the *Click Me* Twine stories were analysed, in different ways. As detailed in Chapter 3, materiality was at the core of the *Click Me* research through the technological writing tool, Twine, but also through the narratives that were produced. Materiality was positioned in the forefront through the writing prompts offered to authors in the *Click Me* Twine module. Both the free writing prompt and the final illness narrative prompt intentionally call on authors to centre their embodied, rather than conceptual, experience of the disease and to think about sensory perception. These prompts ask the authors to write about how it feels to live in a body that is ill by turning to the sensorial experiences of the material body. Narratives produced by the *Click Me* authors tended to foreground the materiality of the body through narrative as a result.

One of the methodological prompts used in the analysis of the *Click Me* data calls on the researcher to consider how the narrative builds the discursive object. This research found a single, common discursive object built into every *Click Me* author's narrative: the abnormal body. Considering the centring of the material body in the writing prompt, body-focused narratives were expected. However, the theme of abnormality of the body was widespread. The abnormal body was written about by authors in both explicit and abstract ways. First, authors wrote about the abnormal body as uncontrollable and requiring control. These narrative framings included the body as uncomfortable and as not adhering to a standard of femininity. The illness of the body was written about as the source of the abnormality but in contrasting ways. Some narratives framed abnormality as inherently a part of the self while others positioned it as an external force acting on the body. Second, authors wrote about the abnormal body in relation to the labour of maintaining normative femininity. These narratives included a sense of being trapped in a circuit, or loop, of maintaining femininity through tedious, relentless rituals on the body.

Third, the *Click Me* narratives wrote about the abnormal body as requiring a cure. This cure, for authors, was framed as an objective they were attempting to achieve by exploring every possible path. Fourth, authors wrote about first discovering the abnormality of the body through a similar narrative scene: the first menstruation. *Click Me* authors discussed recognizing their first period as not behaving the way they believed it should, and therefore making a discovery that their body was abnormal. This moment in adolescence was tied to a theme of childhood sexuality as well. Narratives framed childhood sexuality as something that can be imposed by adults but cannot be discovered by the child on their own. Fifth, authors wrote about a dualized abnormality where the abnormality of the body is linked to either emotional bankruptcy or a Queer identity. Finally, *Click Me* narratives framed the abnormal body as a mystery that requires deciphering. To unravel the mystery of the abnormal body, for authors, ultimately relinquishes guilt where the abnormality is not the fault of the author but the fault of the illness.

Considering how broader discourses shaped and layered onto the narratives, several distinct themes emerged, including relationality, healthcare experience and empowerment. Relationships written about by the *Click Me* authors in their narratives tended to fall into specific categories: the mother, the sister and romantic relationships. The mother was the most frequently coded relationship in the *Click Me* research. Authors wrote about the mother in distinct ways. First, there was a common theme of shame in revealing the abnormality of the body to the mother. This shame was linked, at times, to the first menstruation scene where authors wrote about both a fear and an inevitable duty to disclose the abnormal menstruation to the mother. Second, some *Click Me* narratives constructed a belief system that it is the mother's role to monitor/intervene/maintain the normality of the daughter's body. Third, the *Click Me* narratives included ample discussion around the fear of becoming your mother. Fourth, and similarly, authors discussed fears about not becoming a mother at all. Chapter 5 considers the construction of the mother in the *Click Me* narratives and considers implications for the potential of internalized misogyny through the ways in which the mother is culturally positioned to be at fault for a "dysfunction" of the child's body in ways other parents may not be.

Other relationships that were strongly coded in the *Click Me* research include the sister and the romantic partner. The sister was narratively framed as a symbolic concept, rather than a literal sibling, of a feminine ideal that the illness of hyperandrogenism prevents the author from achieving. Romantic relationships were written about by authors in varying ways. Authors discussed feeling as if the disease of hyperandrogenism strips them of femininity and therefore renders them undesirable to romantic partners. In longer-term heterosexual relationships, authors wrote about feeling as if they are failing in their role of womanhood, a role that is required of them in a romantic partnership. Finally, there was ample discussion in the Twines of moments of unsupportive actions from a romantic partner in contrast to the partner acting as the sole, safe companion to discuss anxieties and fears regarding the illness.

The ways in which larger discourses came to layer onto the *Click Me* narratives emerged through the framing of the healthcare experience as well. Authors, overwhelmingly, framed their experiences in the healthcare system as negative, mainly through feeling subjugated, dehumanized, or dismissed by their physicians or perceiving the physician to lack knowledge on the topic of PCOS or hyperandrogenism. Narratives shared a theme of experiences of violation during particular medical procedures, mainly transvaginal ultrasounds. Authors wrote about either perceiving the procedure as invasive or else not being adequately informed of the various steps. Negative healthcare experiences were positioned by some *Click Me* authors through a lens of intersectionality and discussions of how identity impacts negative healthcare outcomes (specifically discussions around fat bodies, race and gender identity). Finally, some authors discussed unique experiences in a privatized healthcare system through navigating the impacts of capitalism and insurance. Negative healthcare experiences were juxtaposed by authors with what they deemed as positive experiences. Positive healthcare encounters, for the *Click Me* authors, were indicated by feeling validated, heard and understood by clinicians.

Finally, the authors constructed a level of gender dynamics in their stories. There was a sustained belief from the *Click Me* authors that a male physician tended to be present in negative healthcare encounters whereas a female physician may facilitate positive experiences. Positive healthcare encounters were expanded on by authors to include the realm of alternative medicine and alternative approaches to illness. Narratives that framed alternative approaches to illness as beneficial tended to resist grappling with quantitative results. Rather than consider if alternative responses to illness "work" in the sense that they produce a measurable reduction of physical symptoms, these stories tended to assert that alternative practices "work" because they allow the author to feel heard, understood and validated.

The final narrative category identified in the *Click Me* Twines was empowerment. Authors wrote about empowerment in various ways, including how knowledge, diagnosis, and insight can be empowering, and may facilitate transformation and community building. First, the *Click Me* narratives position a formal diagnosis of a disease as political. Increased knowledge of the disease was discussed as empowering the author in a way that emboldens them to extend that power to those around them experiencing similar oppression. Other authors complicated the idea that a formal diagnosis was an inherent resolution. These stories suggest that diagnosis may afford clarity in some respects, but, as a result, further questions emerge. For example, having a formal diagnosis may assist a patient in receiving treatment or navigating the healthcare system, however, *Click Me* authors noted a risk of harm in diagnostic labels as well. Second, the *Click Me* stories tended to conclude on an uplifting note. This narrative ending typically looked like the author undergoing a mindset transformation in order to ultimately accept living with the disease, rather than receiving a cure. Third, empowerment was written about by authors as community-building. The *Click Me* narratives, supported by insight from closing interviews, validated a sense of power that stems from finding kinship with other women and individuals with hyperandrogenism and through support from loved ones.

One of the most compelling findings of this project was the ways in which subject positions formed and how these positions enact or restrict moments for action. All of the *Click Me* narratives used a first-person point of view. Chapter 5 discussed how the literature on literary hypertext considers how conventional Twine games appear to foreground the choices of the reader through the second-person point of view. The *Click Me* narratives, by contrast, centre the subjectivity of the author. This finding does not, however, support claims regarding the game-ness or narrative-ness of the *Click Me* Twines due to the first-person perspective. As the literature on literary hypertext suggests, making structuralist assumptions of game versus narrative erases the complex nuance of writing in hypertext. Notably, perhaps, these are stories and games and interactive fiction and pedagogical tools and therapy—all in one.

Further, the *Click Me* narratives build a formulaic trajectory for the author's agency where the story begins with a lack of agency for the author and, as the narrative progresses, the author is granted or restricted agency through their narrative encounters with other subjects, objects and forces. This phenomenon was found to be important because the authors did not frame the inherent embodiment of hyperandrogenism as restricting agency but as the ways in which illness is taken up culturally. Narratives resisted cultivating moments of granting action for the author through alleviating symptoms of the illness and embraced this action through encounters with cultural forces that pushed back against illness stigma.

In Chapter 5, the process of situating the narrative themes was concluded by an analysis of what is affirmed and erased by the *Click Me* stories and why. In the end, what is affirmed through the analysis of the discursive framing of the narratives is a collective assumption that a female body that experiences masculinizing symptoms is abnormal. This abnormality renders the body in need of control, deciphering and strenuous labour. The dysfunction of the body has the potential to infect the author's psyche as well, resulting in emotional bankruptcy. This belief was present in the inverse as well where emotional bankruptcy is present first and leads to the disruption of the normal functioning of the body. The *Click Me* narratives affirm that bodily abnormality is undesirable because of its relationality with outside agents rather than an inherent undesirability. It is in the *Click Me* author's encounters with other people, institutions and social systems that render their bodies undesirable, rather than the neutral embodiment of symptoms. The *Click Me* narratives, then, position disease as a personal journey. This journey centres the concept of growth where healing is rooted in resolving emotional bankruptcy, gaining knowledge, receiving a formal diagnosis and locating a community of support.

Finally, the *Click Me* narratives collectively assert that encounters in the normative healthcare system are generally dehumanizing, subjugating or violating. The development of gender dynamics is relevant in this belief system where narratives position females over male physicians as more inclined to produce positive healthcare experiences. Ultimately, authors affirm alternative medicine and alternative approaches to illness as effective responses to illness, not because of a measured reduction of symptoms, but because of producing a greater sense of well-being. The collective affirmation of particular beliefs in the *Click Me* narratives is in line with the erasure of counter-discourses including traditional biomedical approaches, a sense of contentment with the abnormal, and questioning the category of abnormality.

In Chapter 6, the ways in which authors employed the digital features of the Twine software to build their narratives were analysed through the context of power relations. Overwhelmingly, the *Click Me* authors believed that the Twine software was user-friendly and straightforward to learn when following the steps outlined in the module. However, this accessibility of the technology was predicated on the assumption of time to concentrate on the module instructions and the emotional or mental capacity to write about difficult experiences. Authors discussed this notion of capacity in different ways. For example, some authors noted that Twine initially felt daunting to learn before they began the module. One *Click Me* author noted that the Twine module was important because it allowed them to complete the storyboard outline before starting the Twine tutorial. This allowed the author to focus on learning the program without being overwhelmed with brainstorming a narrative topic at the same time. Another author explained that the structure of building a Twine story was less overwhelming than writing a narrative on a physical sheet of paper because it breaks the writing process down into manageable sections. While most authors felt prepared to complete the study through online pedagogy, one author felt they would be more successful learning the program in person.

Chapter 6 explores how the digital features of the Click Me narratives—including code—have been shaped by and have responded to broader social forces. Generally, authors chose to incorporate colour, alignment, size and text style codes that contributed to the meaning-making of their Twine stories, in different ways. When the default background colour of the Twines was altered, it was most commonly changed to a standard white background with black text, suggesting that rather than challenge assumed expectations around how a digital narrative document should look, authors chose to reproduce this. Several *Click Me* authors chose to include images in their Twines that generated different meanings. Finally, style codes transformed narratives into a visual experience where the colour, size, style and spacing of the text produced narrative signification. The signification generated from the manipulation of style codes in these narratives cannot be summarised into a general theme or pattern. Each of the narratives in the study incorporated, or chose not to include, style codes that worked to build on the specific connotations of their individual story. This meaning-making process for each narrative, is of course, highly subjective.

Multimodality, specifically choices made to construct the hypertext links, shaped the narrative meaning in various ways for the *Click Me* Twines. The text chosen to be hyperlinks in the stories is significant because the hyperlink is set apart from the bulk of the other text and embodies emphasis. Further, a weaving path was the dominant story structure choice. Authors tended to utilize a weaving path, and at times multiple paths, to design a narrative loop that brings the reader/player back to engage with a previous passage in order to personify the experience of their illness. Using a weaving path to play with the idea of reader choice was a popular strategy for authors in different ways. Some *Click Me* authors designed an illusion of choice while other authors foregrounded the agency of the reader/player. In general, authors employed dead-end linking in various passages of their narrative to create a sense of a lack of options where the only path forward is to move backwards. A strategy, or accident, of a passage with no hyperlink access, added an additional layer of meaning to several stories. For example, a passage with no hyperlink that does not appear to be the "true" end of the narrative creates a sense of stagnation or lack of options to move forward in the narrative.

The *Click Me* Twines most commonly utilized navigational linking. The use of this linking strategy produced a feeling that the reader/player is navigating the story as if it were a space. Navigational linking was also used for knowledge dissemination by designing a Twine that acts as a spatial database of information. The waiting room was the dominant thematic space depicted, and through navigational linking, this room explored themes of anxiety around the healthcare encounter as well as feeling intentionally kept in the dark regarding the nature of the illness. Finally, passages in the *Click Me* Twines were predominately a unified construction, which suggests an affinity with narrative-ness over game-ness, however, literary hypertext scholars such as Salter and Moulthrop argue against this essentialism.

What we come away with here, in Chapter 6, is that the *Click Me* authors used the digital features of the literary hypertext software to structurally chart the narrative of their illness in ways that the author perceived as most conducive to personal reflection. Authors explored the concept of using Twine to visually map out their experiences, and manually organize them by hyperlinking passages, to find a structure that was best suited for therapeutic reflection. This visual map was discussed in different ways by authors including mirroring the human thought process, matching the experience of an illness diagnosis, conveying the feeling of a negative mental health circuit or facilitating personal discoveries through the practice of hyperlinking. Ultimately, authors reflected on the capabilities of Twine through the lens of intersectionality. Authors spoke about the software allowing for the deconstruction and reconstruction of the "web of our identity," or in other words, a way to visually contend with the array of identities that produce the self. Twine has a sociohistorical legacy as a tool of resistance for those pushed to the margins of game development, but the *Click Me* authors highlight the real-life ways in which power relations monopolize capacity, particularly the capacity to sit down and learn a new technology for writing.

The key findings discussed above come to a pivotal moment at the central question of the effectiveness of literary hypertext as a tool for women and nonbinary individuals to write illness narratives that construct positive relationships between themselves and the world. The *Click Me* authors reiterated the same belief that writing a single illness narrative, in any format, cannot "cure" or "fix" the self. The value, for authors, in engaging in writing a literary hypertext illness narrative was found through the facilitation of reflection on past experiences. This reflection was discussed by authors in various ways including leading to new vantage points to better understand emotions, establishing a deeper connection to the self, and validating past experiences of injustice. Ultimately, authors come to a conclusion that reintroduces the value of narrative medicine. For literary hypertext illness narratives to cultivate true therapeutic value, according to the *Click Me* authors, they should be used as a tool, not only by the author to reflect on experience but also for the wider, social and medical community to read and learn about the experience of hyperandrogenism.

## Impact and Contribution

The *Click Me* research discussed in this book is a critical piece of a larger, complex puzzle of research taking place at the intersection of medical/health humanities, digital humanities and gender studies. It responds to a query in these fields that is grappling with novel, innovative approaches to responding to sex-based illness. The findings, discussed above, are important for a cultural moment that is embracing digital connectivity while calling awareness to the limitations of normative approaches to illness. Ultimately, what we come away with is aligned with the second-wave scholarship on literary hypertext that cautions against an over-enthusiastic proclamation of the revolutionary capabilities of the medium. In response to the scholarship that challenges the claims of the inherent narrative self, this book assumes literary hypertext illness narratives as one potentially beneficial approach to responding to illness rather than the only path. Significantly, the intention of this book is to bring to the forefront a specific corpus and research topic that is fresh to the academic literature and, critically, to public discourse. At the date this book was written, there is no research published on the effectiveness of literary hypertext as a tool to write illness narratives for marginalized people. Further, representation of the experiences of women and nonbinary individuals with hyperandrogenism in academic literature is scarce. This book is intended to be a first step to aid subsequent research on the topic of literary hypertext illness narratives and the lived experience of hyperandrogenism, both in their intersection and independently.

Like Twine, the impact of the *Click Me* research, in particular, is branching and forging multiple paths. First, this book has outlined a novel approach to theorizing the experience of hyperandrogenism. The theorizing of the construction of the abnormal body through the narratives of individuals with hyperandrogenism is a completely novel and critical contribution to the literature. We desperately need to hear the voices of women and individuals with hyperandrogenism to understand their experiences of pathologization, ultimately to inform the development of more ethical approaches to healthcare. This book champions this cause.

Second, the findings of this book hope to innovate the practice of therapeutic illness narratives for marginalized individuals. The *Click Me* research contributes to a larger discussion around access to alternative methods for responding to illness, particularly for marginalized identities. The information in this book can support individuals in accessing literary hypertext software and writing illness narratives online. Chapter 4 outlines the unique development of a Twine module design informed by a political narrative therapy framework. Organizations can utilize the findings detailed throughout this chapter to develop literary hypertext modules of their own to facilitate illness narrative writing for their communities. These organizations may look like illness advocacy groups, schools or illness support communities.

Third, this book presents an innovative proposal to address the sociopolitical marginalization of hyperandrogenism in the treatment of the illness, through the application of narrative medicine. This proposal calls for educating healthcare providers and the public on the political experience of hyperandrogenism in ways that moves through, alongside and outside institutional walls. What this might look like is nuanced: perhaps advocating for the inclusion of person-centred experiences of hyperandrogenism in medical school classrooms, while also investing in internet access in rural areas so marginalized individuals can share their stories online in their own words. In considering this nuanced call, I wonder what it would look like to prescribe a Twine illness narrative in the treatment of hyperandrogenism. How could Twine illness narratives be incorporated into patient digital files for clinicians to learn from? How can we provide a suite of access to narrative therapy or illness narratives in ways that offer the option for the patient to sit in the driver's seat. In other words, where do we start?

**Recommendations for Future Research**

Understanding the limitations of the findings of this book allows for targeted recommendations for future research to fill important gaps. Critical research to build on this project would consider studying the benefits of literary hypertext illness narratives for people with hyperandrogenism with a larger participant pool. A project like this would require ample funding. Similarly, altering the facilitation design method of this study in future related research would produce helpful data. This may look like incorporating in-person Twine workshops to teach literary hypertext illness narratives instead of, or to supplement, the module. Additionally, researching various application methods and environments would contribute to relevant data on the topic, including the facilitation of literary hypertext illness narrative workshops in therapy settings, schools or the clinical context. Finally, limitations of the methodology, including turning to frameworks that can capture the decision-making process for code and digital design choices made by authors would supplement the project of this book.

Branching expansively from this project would see a two-fold scholarly focus: research on other digital technologies for writing literary hypertext illness narratives and centring other pathologized identities. This book centres hyperandrogenism, however, the study of this disease in particular opened up paths to consider an array of varying embodiments and pathologized identities in relation to illness narratives including identities of disability, DSD, and neurodiversity. There is a mountain of progress required to understand the experiences of these embodiments in both academic literature and our sociocultural discourse. Further, this book resists valorizing a particular technology like Twine, or even a genre of writing like literary hypertext, as the only/best method for illness narratives. I am interested in expanding conceptualizations of what coping with illness can look like and how the digital space is opening new doors for healing, resisting and finding community. Subsequent research to build on this project, then, would consider telling the story of illness through other digital practices such as social media, comment sections, games, code, film, video conferencing, etc. For example, in 2022, Astrid Ensslin and I published "The Possibilities of Illness Narratives in Virtual Reality for Bodies at the Margins" in the journal of *Digital Creativity*. In this article, we look at how VR technology may be utilized as a method for illness narrative creation for pathologized identities. Pushing the research in a direction curious of what else can be discovered in the digital space is the intention of this project.

**A Final Note on the Impact of Narrative**

This chapter began with an outline of the key findings of this research project related to matter and feminist new materialism, narrative themes, contextualization of themes, and technological findings. The following sections outlined the main contributions of this book, the limitations of the *Click Me* research project, and recommendations for future research. Ultimately, this chapter responds to the research question of how literary hypertext can be used as a tool for women and nonbinary individuals to write illness narratives that construct positive relationships between their identities and the world. The *Click Me* authors used literary hypertext software to structurally chart the narrative of their illness in ways most conducive to personal reflection. Authors used the Twine program to visually map out their experiences, and manually organize them by hyperlinking passages, to find a structure that was perceived as best suited for therapeutic reflection. Ultimately, authors believed that writing a single illness narrative, in any format, cannot "cure" or "fix" the self. The value, for authors, in engaging in writing a Twine illness narrative was found through the unique process of reflection on past experiences. Ultimately, the findings of this book return to the framework of narrative medicine. Authors believed that for literary hypertext illness narratives to cultivate true therapeutic value, they would be tools, not only by the author to reflect on experience, but for the wider social and medical community to read and learn about the experience of hyperandrogenism.

I mentioned in an earlier section that this book would end with a note on the impact of narrative. There is such a vast need inside, outside and alongside the normative healthcare system for innovative methods to respond to emotional-based issues related to illness. As a culture, we are simultaneously reckoning with the impacts of COVID-19, increased healthcare costs, diminished healthcare access and insurance coverage, the soaring cost of living, and a general lack of temporal, physical and emotional capacity to tend to our mental health. When our identities devolve into international political fodder and our bodies become incongruent with our *selves*, how do we move forward? I believe, after listening to the *Click Me* authors that the answer is that we move forward by telling our stories. That simple action will beget further progress: improved representation in healthcare, increased funding for hyperandrogenism research, enhanced access to healthcare services, funding for innovative therapeutic tools, and so on. Moving forward, we need to consider how to design paths that open up access to therapy in ways that are intentional, evidence-informed, humanistic and safe. But why don't you tell me, reader, what do you think?

## Works Cited

Amnesty International Canada. "Appalling Anti-Trans Policy Changes in Alberta." *Amnesty International Canada*, 1 February 2024, https://amnesty.ca/human-rights-news/appalling-anti-trans-policy-changes-in-alberta/. Accessed 13 March 2025.

Arizona State Legislature. *Senate Bill 1138*. 55th Leg., 2nd Reg. Sess., 2022, https://www.azleg.gov/legtext/55leg/2R/bills/SB1138S.pdf. Accessed 13 March 2025.

Butler, Judith. *Bodies That Matter: On the Discursive Limits of "Sex"*. Routledge, 2011.

Butler, Judith. *Undoing Gender*. Routledge, 2004, pp. 40–56.
Canguilhem, Georges. *The Normal and the Pathological*. Zone Books, 1991.
Couser, G. Thomas. "Disability, Life Narrative, and Representation." *PMLA*, vol. 120, no. 2, 2005, pp. 602–606.
Couser, G. Thomas. *Recovering Bodies: Illness, Disability, and Life Writing*. University of Wisconsin Press, 1997.
Couser, G. Thomas. *Signifying Bodies: Disability in Contemporary Life Writing*. University of Michigan Press, 2009.
Couser, G. Thomas. *Vulnerable Subjects: Ethics and Life Writing*. Cornell University Press, 2004.
Foucault, Michel. *Discipline and Punish*. Penguin, 1991.
Foucault, Michel. *The History of Sexuality, Vol. II: The Use of Pleasure*. Translated by Robert Hurley, Penguin, 1985.
Frank, Arthur W. *The Wounded Storyteller: Body, Illness, and Ethics*, 2nd ed. The University of Chicago Press, 2013.
Legislative Assembly of Alberta. *Bill 26, the Health Statutes Amendment Act, 2024*. 31st Leg., 1st Sess., 30 May 2023a.
Legislative Assembly of Alberta. *Health Professions Act*. King's Printer. Accessed 13 March 2025.
Legislative Assembly of Alberta. *The Education Amendment Act, 2024* (formerly Bill 27). King's Printer, 30 May 2023b.
Legislative Assembly of Alberta. *The Fairness and Safety in Sport Act*, 2024 (formerly Bill 29). King's Printer, 30 May 2023c.
Perram, Megan, and Astrid Ensslin. "The Possibilities of Illness Narratives in Virtual Reality for Bodies at the Margins." *Digital Creativity*, vol. 33, no. 2, 2022, pp. 128–156.
Semenya, Caster. "Running in a Body That's My Own." *The New York Times*, 21 October 2023. Archived from the original on 28 October 2023. Retrieved 28 October 2023.
Trans Legislation Tracker. *Trans Legislation, 2025*, https://translegislation.com/. Accessed 13 March 2025.

# Index

Pages in *italics* refer to figures, pages in **bold** refer to tables, and pages followed by "n" refer to notes.

Printed in the United States
by Baker & Taylor Publisher Services